The Challenge of Reproductive
Medicine at Catholic Universities

The Challenge of Reproductive Medicine at Catholic Universities

Time to Leave the Catacombs

Edited by
Ivo Brosens

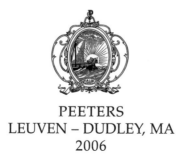

PEETERS
LEUVEN – DUDLEY, MA
2006

Library of Congress Cataloging-in-Publication Data

The challenge of reproductive medicine at Catholic Universities: time to leave the catacombs / [edited by] Ivo Brosens
   p. cm.
   ISBN 90-429-1762-8 (alk. paper)
   1. Reproductive health--Study and teaching--Belgium--Louvain. 2. Catholic universities and colleges--Health promotion services--Belgium--Louvain. 3. Human reproductive technology--Religious aspects--Catholic Church. 4. Birth control--Religious aspects--Catholic Church. 5. Medical ethics--Religious aspects--Catholic Church. 6. Katholieke Universiteit te Leuven (1970-) I. Brosens, I. A.

RG133.C43 2006
618.1'78--dc22

                                             2006041694

© 2006 – Peeters, Bondgenotenlaan 153, B-3000 Leuven – Belgium

D. 2006/0602/54
ISBN-10 90-429-1762-8
ISBN-13 9789042917620

To the memory of Kamiel Vandenberghe, a pioneer in fetomaternal medicine and a man of integrity

TABLE OF CONTENTS

ACKNOWLEDGMENTS

This book has been accomplished by the contribution of many people that were involved in different ways and at different stages of its development. Thanks go to in the first place to Marcel Renaer and Maurice De Wachter for their most crucial contributions which are central in the book. Leading clinicians and researchers including Victoria Jennings, Enrique Oyarzún, Tom Eskes, Jacques Donnez, Jean-Jacques Cassiman and Jan Deprest have contributed to present an anthology of the resarch in reproductive medicine at Catholic universities around the world. The contribution of colleagues for the following sections is greatly acknoweleged: Robert Pijnenborg (I, 3 and 4), Jan Brosens (II, 5), Omer Steeno (VI, 19 and 20), Raul Ruiz Cordoba (IX, 29), Jan Kremer (IX, 29), Ricardo Marana (IX,29), Michael Thomure (IX, 29), Craig Winkel (IX, 29), Michael Zinaman (IX, 29), Marie-Madeleine Dolmans, Dominique Demylle (X, 35), François Luks, Liesbeth Lewi, Roland Devlieger, Dominique van Schoubroeck, Marc Vandevelde and Toni Lerut (X, 37).

Documents on ethical guidelines were kindly provided by professor J. Vermylen (K.U.Leuven), professor P. Spauwen (Radboud University) and professor J.M. Maloteaux (U.C.L.).

Linguistic assistance was provided by Jessica Woodworth.

Paul Peeters, Head of Peeters Publications, and the Peeters production team have been invaluable in turning this project into a unique book.

INTRODUCTION

This book was written in the hope that it may interest those in the Catholic world who care about reproductive health. The first reason was to document the struggle of the many people who have contributed, over a period of more than fifty years, to the development of reproductive medicine at the Catholic University of Leuven (K.U.Leuven) in Belgium. Together with many others at different Catholic universities in the Low Countries, Belgium and Holland, they were instrumental in establishing a modern clinical service that is effective and acceptable for patients, inspired by a Christian vision and, hopefully, compatible with the mission of Catholic universities.

Reproductive medicine is one of the most challenging fields in modern medicine. New technologies, developed at barely believable pace, have profoundly changed many areas of reproductive medicine, including fertility control, infertility treatment, embryology, prenatal diagnosis and fetal surgery. Ethical dilemmas raised by the clinical application of these technologies were addressed at the Catholic universities of the Low Countries through dialogue between physicians, theologians, philosophers, clergymen and many other involved people. Step by step a modern approach to reproductive medicine was developed, inspired by freedom of choice, humanity, and respect for others.

Part 1 of the book discusses the bio-medical background of controversial contemporary issues in reproductive medicine. Modern reproductive medicine started in the 1950s with the discovery that ovulation and menstruation are under the direct control of sex steroid hormones. Safe family planning was at that time a major issue in Western countries. In the 1960s, the two most significant advances in modern contraception occurred – the nearly simultaneous invention of the "pill" and the intrauterine contraceptive device. In 1956, Jacques Ferin, Professor of Gynecologic Endocrinology at the Catholic University of Leuven, discovered a very active progestogenic steroid, called methylestrenolone or lynestrenol, that suppressed ovulation. He was able to show that with lynestrenol a hypo-estrogenic amenorrhoea could be induced in women. In 1958, Louis Janssens, Professor at the Faculty of Theology, discussed in *Ephemerides Theologiae Lovanienses* the question: "L'inhibition de l'ovulation est-elle moralement licite?" Menstruation and ovulation are two fundamental manifestations of reproductive competence, but are they redundant or, as has been suggested, obsolete in the absence of a desire to reproduce? Modern society is increasingly dependent on interventional technologies for reproduction, but have women become less aware of natural fertility signals and are they less able to conceive spontaneously? As the quality of the uterine environment around the time of conception profoundly impacts on the long-term health of the progeny, will the liberal use of assisted reproductive technologies increase the incidence of disease in adult life?

Part 2 of the book describes in detail, and with anecdotes, the history of modern reproductive medicine at the K.U.Leuven. In the 1970s, innovations were made in the treatment of male and female infertility with the introduction of donor insemination, hormones for the induction of ovulation and the microsurgical and endoscopic techniques for reconstructive surgery. In the 1980s, in vitro fertilization and other assisted reproductive technologies revolutionized the treatment of infertility. This is a tale of errors and mistakes and the story has its black pages. However, from the onset, clinical practice was founded on a responsible ethical approach. In two compelling exposés Maurice De Wachter describes how the discipline of personalist ethics was developed and applied to reproductive medicine. This unique period of intense dialogue between the University and Church is remembered by Marcel Renaer, one of the founders of the reproductive services at the K.U.Leuven. During this period the Catholic University of Leuven was, in 1971, split into two separate universities, a Dutch-speaking Katholieke Universiteit van Leuven (K.U.Leuven) and a French-speaking Université Catholique de Louvain (U.C.L.). After 1971 our history continues to describe the developments at the K.U.Leuven.

Part 3 discusses how reproductive medicine is currently practiced at Catholic university hospitals worldwide, especially in the fields of fertility control and infertility treatment. Clinical practice is far from uniform. While academic authorities at most Catholic universities proclaim to follow the Church directives strictly, the physician-patient relationship has remain largely unaffected and outside their control. A clear rift has emerged between progressive and orthodox Catholic universities. This started with the introduction of contraception but the rift widened immensely with the introduction of new reproductive technologies, such as assisted reproductive technologies and prenatal diagnosis. As some progressive Catholic universities have now embraced embryonic stem cell research, even basic medical research risks becoming polarized. Are progressive Catholic universities in the Low Countries silently heading towards a schism in the Catholic world?

The fundamental question that runs throughout this book is whether modern reproductive medicine, based on personalist ethics and practised at progressive Catholic universities, is compatible with the Catholic doctrine. If so, has the time come for these universities to take a stand and leave the catacombs?

Ivo Brosens

PART 1

BIO-MEDICAL CONTEXT

CHAPTER I

SEX AND REPRODUCTION

The physiological events of menstruation, ovulation, gamete transport, fertilization, implantation and placenta formation have been well described in modern medicine. However, the significance of these events is sometimes poorly understood or even distorted to fit an ideology. This chapter discusses briefly some fundamental aspects of human reproduction that are important to understand topics discussed in subsequent chapters.

1. Is menstruation obsolete?

What is menstruation?

Menstruation is a powerful sign of reproductive life. The first menstruation, or the "menarche", is the sign that the ovarian function has started. The link between the ovaries and menstruation was first suspected in 1872 when surgical removal of the ovaries performed in normal women resulted in the suppression of menstruation. One of the first documented effects of the ovarian function on the menstrual cycle was that of the shift in basal body temperature (BBT) as described by van de Velde in 1904 (fig1.1). He meticulously recorded a large amount of data and pointed out that cyclic ovarian changes cause the menstrual rhythm. His observation of the biphasic basal body temperature of the menstruating woman led, many years before the era of hormones, to the conclusion that menstruation does not predict ovulation, but that menstruation is the result of foregoing ovulation.

Today we know that the biphasic basal body temperature chart in menstruating women represents an ovulatory cycle. The postovulatory hyperthermic plateau is an effect of the progesterone secretion by the corpus luteum and reflects the duration of the luteal phase. Therefore, in the anovulatory cycle, when no ovulation occurs and no

Biphasic basal body temperature

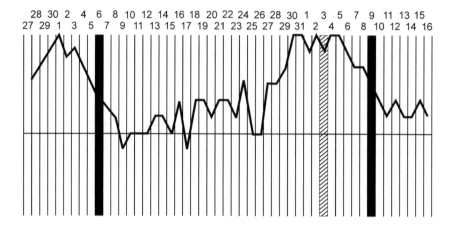

☒ Expected day of menstruation

■ Menstruation

Figure 1.1 Normal menstruation (solid bar) in a 37-year-old woman. The last temperature wave lasted longer than normal. Also the menstrual bleeding occurred later than expected (striped bar).
Modified after Th. H. van de Velde (1904) Ueber den Zusammenhang zwischen Ovarialfunktion, Wellenbewegung un Menstrualblutung und ueber die Enstehung des sogenannten Mittelschmerzes.

progesterone is produced, the basal body temperature chart remains monophasic.

The old belief that menstruation was a sign of fertility was no longer tenable. Somebody described menstruation plastically as "the bloody tears of the uterus that failed to become pregnant".

The natural variation in the menstrual cycle

In 1967, the reproductive anthropologist, Alan Treloar, published a study of the natural variation that occurs in the human menstrual cycle. The study was based not on personal opinion but on the statistical analysis of scientific recordings of data in an unselected population. With the introduction of oral contraceptives, such a study would no longer be possible. Treloar began the prospective study

Variability in duration
of menstrual cycle

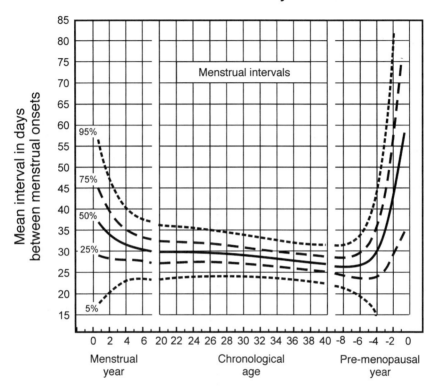

Figure 1.2 Normal curve contours for the distribution of the length of the menstrual cycle in three zones of experience. Modified after Treloar (1967).

in 1933 and invited schoolgirls and student nurses, and later their own children, to participate in the study. They collected precious information on the intra-person variation in menstrual interval over a total of 22.754 calendar years of experience. The study was published in 1967 and some of the conclusions were remarkable (fig 1.2).

- There is no substantial evidence for the widely held belief that women normally vary in menstrual interval about a value of 28 days common to all.
- Complete regularity in menstruation over a long period of time is a myth.

- With regard to menstrual interval, there are three zones in menstrual life: the first few years (post-menarche), a mid-life zone from 20 to 40 years, and the last few years (pre-menopause).
- All menstrual histories show individualities.

The paper firmly established that each woman has her own central trend and variation, both of which change with age.

When is menstruation a disease?

Although menstruation is usually felt to be a natural and physiological occurrence to which most women accommodate without complaint and with scarcely visible impact on their daily lives, the majority nonetheless experience low-level discomfort, such as bloating, fatigue, breast tension and backache in the week before their periods. For about one-third of the female population, the premenstrual symptoms they experience during this time can cause significant discomfort.

Moreover, some 5 % of women suffer from the so-called premenstrual syndrome (PMS) with difficult bouts of emotional upheaval including fear, frustration and rage that can have devastating effects on a woman's daily life. The most severe symptoms are fatigue, irritability, abdominal distension, nervous tension, breast tenderness, mood changes, depression, increased appetite and sleep disturbance or insomnia.

Today, premenstrual discomfort, and particularly PMS, need not be accepted as inevitable. Symptomatic relief is the most frequent treatment and a great variety of medications such as diuretics, vitamins B6 and E, tranquillizers and antidepressants have been prescribed. The most effective treatment, however, is ovulation suppression, which prevents the hormonal fluctuations in the early stage in the menstrual cycle. It is a logical approach for resolving premenstrual discomfort and PMS at its origin.

Several disruptive disorders can occur during the periods of menstruation. Dysmenorrhea is the most common disorder and is more common in young women, particularly adolescents. Most women can obtain relief with the use of aspirin or non-steroidal anti-inflammatory products while oral contraceptive pills can control severe dysmenorrhea by eliminating the true menstruation.

The uterine bleeding associated with the cyclical use of oral contraceptive pills causes the most regular menstrual bleeding because it is not dependent on ovarian activity. It has aptly been referred to as a withdrawal bleeding or pseudo-menstruation because it is actually a simulation of the real physiological event. Instead of spontaneous menstruation, women using the pill experience a withdrawal bleeding due to an abrupt drop in the level of the pill hormones. The bleeding represents the shedding of the endometrial layers that have been affected by the hormones.

The influences of a modern lifestyle

Changes in modern society have greatly influenced the nature of human reproduction. In modern societies the gradual changes with earlier age at menarche, later first pregnancies, fewer term pregnancies, much shorter durations of lactation and perhaps a slightly later menopause mean that a woman in modern industrialized society will experience several hundred more menstrual cycles in a lifetime than her more primitive forebears, perhaps some four hundred and fifty as compared with one hundred. This means that the uterus is exposed to multiple, regular, major fluctuations in hormones every month in a way that is likely to encourage growth of uterine tissue and even tumor formation of these tissues in women who are genetically predisposed. In addition, there are few full-term pregnancies and short or no lactation periods to provide a measure of protection against these growths.

In comparative reproductive biology there is evidence that higher primates that are prevented from becoming pregnant have a much greater chance of developing pathology like endometriosis and myomatous nodules of the uterus. Anthropological studies have also contributed to a growing body of evidence that women's bodies were designed by natural selection to spend most of the time in lactation-associated amenorrhea. These studies add support to the view that hormonal contraceptives can be made safer if they forego the hormonal swings associated with menstruation. This conclusion is further reinforced by evidence that menstrual bleeding serves no adaptive purpose.

Endometriosis a modern disease

Endometriosis is one of the most common diseases in women of reproductive age. The disease causes chronic pelvic pain, infertility and ovarian cysts and the risk is greatest among nulliparous women with earlier age at menarche and shorter menstrual cycles, while among parous women the risk is decreased with parity and lifetime duration of lactation.

The disease is characterized by the presence of small implants of endometrium-like tissue outside the uterine cavity and, unfortunately, is frequently diagnosed at a late stage after many years of unexplained pain or persisting infertility.

Endometriosis caused by menstruation

It is usually not realized that at menstruation the endometrial debris is eliminated not only through the lower genital tract, but also through the Fallopian tubes into the peritoneal cavity (fig 1.3). Much of the debris in the peritoneal cavity is cleared by the immune cell system, but healthy endometrial fragments can implant on the peritoneal membrane or on the peritoneal surface of intra-abdominal organs such as the ovaries, the bowel or bladder.

While endometrial regurgitation into the peritoneal cavity is a normal phenomenon in menstruating women, some 5–10% of women

Retrograde menstruation

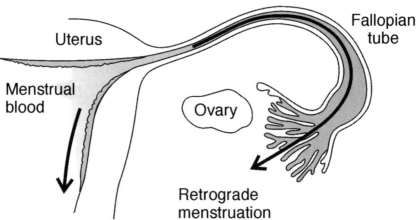

Figure 1.3 At menstruation, the endometrial debris is eliminated not only through the lower genital tract, but also through the Fallopian tubes into the peritoneal cavity.

develop the disease endometriosis. The question arises: why do not all menstruating women develop the disease endometriosis? It is hypothesized that in most women the normal peritoneal defense mechanisms protect against the development of the disease, but in some women there may be an excess of retrograde menstruation that cannot be cleared, while in others the immune system may fail to remove the menstrual debris.

Endometriosis is likely to be a modern disease, although an American historian recently argued that the disease was described in late seventeenth- and eighteenth-century dissertations presented at European universities.

Endometriosis; a disease because it is bleeding

The disease endometriosis can severely affect the sexual and reproductive life of young women by causing dysmenorrhea, discomfort and pain during sexual intercourse and pain at defecation, particularly during menstruation.

The endometriotic implants respond similarly to, but more irregularly than the endometrium in the uterus to the ovarian hormones by bleeding and develop painful, hemorrhagic and inflammatory nodules in pelvic structures. At the site of the ovary, the bleeding and the adhesions on the surface of the ovary form so-called chocolate cysts, which have the structure of a pseudo-uterus with a cavity lined by endometrial-like tissue. Ovarian chocolate cysts, however, are not painful and are frequently detected in young asymptomatic women at the time of an ultrasound examination of the pelvis, for example, during infertility investigation.

A well-known example is the tragic history Marilyn Monroe. She might have looked glamorous but for much of her life Marilyn Monroe endured chronic pains and reproductive failures. She married at the age of 26 and her sex life was affected by dyspareunia. Surgery failed. The marriage broke down after four years. Her modeling career was constantly interrupted by severe dysmenorrhea. Surgery for ovarian endometrioma also failed. Her desire for children in her second marriage ended in an ectopic pregnancy and miscarriage. Surgery failed again. Between 1952 and 1962, the year she died at the age of 36, she had in total six abdominal surgeries related to endometriosis, pain and infertility. She became addicted to painkillers, which eventually played a part in her death. This tragic story illustrates how severe endometriosis can result, in many cases, in extensive pelvic lesions,

adhesions and distorsion of the pelvic anatomy, which are a cause of chronic
pelvic pains, infertility and repeat surgeries.

The gynecologist who pioneered the development of oral contraceptives
and understood its potential use in gynecologic disorders like endometrio-
sis, practiced in nearby Westwood, where Marilyn moved to live in 1961,
and he had many Hollywood stars among his patients. Marilyn Monroe was
not one of them. Ironically, the injectable hormone, DepoProvera^R, which
inhibits ovulation and menstruation and is very effective in severe
endometriosis, was discovered a year after Marilyn's death. Other hormone
products to treat endometriosis were introduced in the 1970s and 1980s.
They were all based on suppressing ovulation and menstruation.

Natural and abnormal suppression of menstruation

During the so-called reproductive period, usually considered
between 15 and 45 years of age, women often stop menstruating naturally due to pregnancy and lactation. With high fertility and long
lactation, therefore, the number of times that a woman actually experiences menstruation can be dramatically curtailed. There are also
other circumstances such as physical exercise and diet that can
reduce the number of menstruations in a woman's lifetime.

The suppression of menstruation per se is not a risk for a woman's
health. However, the absence of menstruation in women of reproductive age is considered a sign of disease and should be investigated as an abnormality if the woman is neither pregnant, breast-
feeding nor under ovarian steroid hormone suppressing therapy.
There are several conditions where the absence of menstruation is a
symptom, but not the underlying cause of the disease process. Treatment to artificially restore a simulated pattern of menstrual flow does
nothing to resolve the underlying disease process or the main problem, which is usually infertility. In fact, maintenance of amenorrhea
until it is possible to restore ovulation can be beneficial.

Surveys undertaken in the 1970s and 1980s suggested that suppression of menstruation or amenorrhea was unacceptable to most
women. More recent research done by the University of Edinburgh
suggests that increasing numbers of women in the developed world
would prefer to menstruate less often. In a questionnaire survey of
over 1000 women attending family-planning clinics and 290 contraceptive providers in China, South Africa, Nigeria and Scotland, only
among black women in Africa did the majority like having periods.

In all other groups, most women disliked the periods, which were "inconvenient" and associated with menstrual problems. Given the choice, the majority would opt to bleed only once every three months, or not at all.

2. The fertility window and fertility awareness

Sexual intercourse is unlikely to result in conception unless it occurs during the six-day fertile interval ending on the day of ovulation. Using natural fertility methods the epidemiologist Allen Wilcox found, in 1995, that among healthy women trying to conceive, nearly all pregnancies can be attributed to intercourse during a six-day period ending on the day of ovulation. During this period the cervical mucus is an important biological marker for the self-determination of the fertile period.

Vulvar observations

The vulvar mucus changes were described by Billings in 1972 as the so-called 'ovulation method of natural family planning'. The method teaches women how to interpret the vaginal discharges of mucus during the menstrual cycle and is one of the natural family planning methods.

The daily mucus observations are classified according to their feeling and appearance, ranging from a score of 1 (no discharge and dry) to 4 (transparent, stretchy and slippery). The mucus reaches a high score before ovulation.

The characteristic changes in vaginal discharges, which occur during the menstrual cycle, are caused by the mucus secretion of the glands in the endocervical canal (fig 2.1). The production of the transparent, stretchy and slippery mucus results from the rise of estrogens, which are produced by the pre-ovulatory follicle. The role of the estrogenic mucus is to enhance progressive sperm motility and to allow for penetration, storage and transport of normal spermatozoa. The properties of cervical mucus determine whether sperms will be capable of penetration and survival and of being transported to the Fallopian tube, where the fertilization of the egg by the sperm occurs. The progesterone produced at the time of ovulation and during the luteal phase exerts a strong anti-estrogenic effect and under its influ-

Sperm transport at peak mucus day

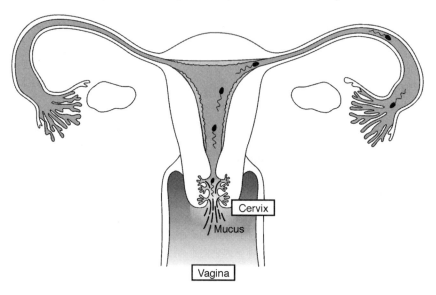

Figure 2.1 On the peak day or the day before ovulation the cervical canal is open and the mucus is very fluid allowing easy passage of the spermatozoa.

ence the mucus becomes thick and sticky and blocks penetration by spermatozoa.

In the past the mucus method has received bad publicity due to the dogmatic claims that were made by the inventor of the method. The literature advocating the use of the method did not supply the scientific data on the efficacy of the method in unselected populations. The method was promoted by ideological arguments and dismissed and incriminated other methods of family planning. The website of the Billings ovulation method refers to an article by Dr. Billings written in 1996 on "Couple's Infertility: Scientific Value and Human Richness of the Billings Method". It is staggering to read the conclusion that the method is "to be accepted as the primary management of infertility, *no matter what other disorders may be contributory*" or "For the majority of couples who have had difficulty in achieving conception *no other course of action is necessary beyond the competent instruction of the woman regarding the cervical mucus pattern and encouragement to keep daily record*". The unscientific statements were far from promoting the true value of the method and, on the contrary, casted doubt on the benefits of the method, antagonized scientists and clinicians and polarized public opinion.

The fertility window

Recent studies by WHO have shown that, in women with regular cycles varying between 26 and 32 days, no pregnancy occurs with intercourse before day 8 or after day 19, when one starts counting the first day of menstruation as day one. However, within this period of 12 days the probability of pregnancy varies from 1% to 40%.

Using vulvar mucus observations, scientists from the National Institute of Environmental Health Sciences and Georgetown University were able to show that the duration of this fertile window is not more than six days when fertihty is defined as the probability that intercourse results in pregnancy at a rate greater than 5%. The mucus characteristics predict the day-specific probabilities of conception

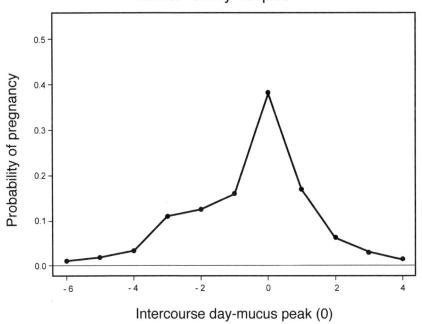

Figure 2.2 Probability of pregnancy from intercourse on a single day in the menstrual cycle relative to the peak mucus day for normally fertile couples. After Stanford et al. 2003

within the fertile interval and the highest probability of pregnancy. This probability increases dramatically to nearly 40% on the peak day of vulvar mucus for normally fertile couples (fig 2.2).

Regardless of the timing of intercourse relative to ovulation, pregnancy probabilities are highest when vulvar observations indicate the presence of the most fertile-type estrogenic mucus. Hence the vulvar observations of cervical mucus predict not only the fertile days of the cycle, or the fertility window, but also the probabilities of conception within the fertile interval. Moreover, with age there is no change of the vulvar mucus in fertile women.

The monitoring of the mucus provides important and additional information not provided by other methods for identifying the fertility window. In particular, methods based on cycle monitoring by daily vaginal ultrasound and/or urinary luteinization hormone (LH) detection are not informative about the probability of conception at a particular time during the fertile interval within an ovulatory cycle

Association between conception and mucus vs ovulation day

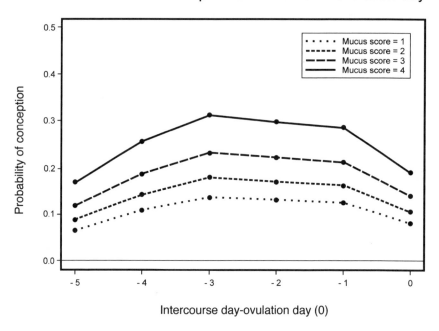

Figure 2.3 Estimated probability of pregnancy with a single act of intercourse in the fertile interval conditional on mucus observations. (Bigelow et al. 2004)

(fig 2.3). In addition, such monitoring is expensive and inconvenient and can miss the beginning of the fertile interval. Hence, scientific data have documented that self-observation of vulvar mucus provides a useful biological marker of days with high conception probabilities.

There is now increasing evidence that the self-observation and monitoring of the vulvar mucus is an efficient and safe method for achieving conception as well as family planning. In Chapter X, Victoria Jennings describes the recent advances in the use of the mucus method for family planning. Teaching fertility awareness should be part of every sex and reproduction educational program. Once a woman intends to become pregnant, knowledge of vulvar mucus changes is likely to give her confidence in her fertility capacity and expedite early conception. Accurate information on methods for effective conception is no less important than the information on effective contraception.

Yolanda was a 47-year-old social worker who married at the age of 40 years. For many years she had been taking care of her sick mother. She doubted whether at her age she could still have a child, but the inner urge continued to return. Last year she had a cardiac check-up and everything was fine. Her menstrual pattern was normal, although the menstruations were less than before. This year she had a delay of menstruation, but the pregnancy test was negative. She was undecided whether to try to become pregnant or let it happen. As a social worker she was well informed about the risks of mongolism. She apparently decided to try to become pregnant after I had explained the risks. I also explained to the mucus method her to identify the fertility window, and advised her to take the afternoon off with her husband on the peak mucus day and have a lovely dinner in the early evening when she was likely to ovulate. Her husband was four years younger, and for this reason it would also be advantageous to plan sexual intercourse on the peak mucus day. If she was still fertile she would have a good chance to conceive within the next six months. She had to confess that she had never heard about the method.

Benefits of fertility awareness

There are many benefits of using fertility awareness methods for couples attempting to conceive.

Firstly, knowledge of the fertile period and the use of the peak fertility day for the timing of intercourse enable the woman to maximize the chance of conception and to avoid unnecessary and worrisome delays. Recently, it has been shown that, as in other mammals, there is in the human a co-ordination of intercourse with ovulation. The frequency rises during the follicular phase, peaking at ovulation and declining abruptly thereafter. It is, hence, unlikely that the timing of intercourse by a fertility awareness method is causing stress. In contrast, the current recommendation of sexual intercourse every two or three days to optimize the chance of pregnancy is more likely to be a continuous cause of stress for the couple. In some women, the stress caused by a fear of infertility may cause ovarian dysfunction, thereby contributing to the delay in conception.

Secondly, the timing of intercourse to the peak fertility day improves the chance of pregnancy in couples with fertility problems. In unexplained infertility, the duration of the fertile window, or days with a likelihood of conception greater than 5%, is not more than three days. The knowledge of these days allows the planning of intercourse during this short but most fertile period of the menstrual cycle. From a male perspective, the cervical mucus vitally regulates sperm survival and transport through the reproductive tract. In a prospective study involving seven European family planning centers, 782 couples recorded daily if they had intercourse and the nature of cervical mucus. It was found that on those days where cervical mucus was not evident, intercourse was 50% less successful with partners in their late 30s and early 40s when compared with younger age groups. When secretions were more conducive for sperm transport, the effect of male age diminishes steadily from 21% on days with damp secretions to 11% on days with thick mucus, and finally to only 4% on days with the most fertile-type mucus. Therefore, the effect of male age on fecundity can be minimized by timing intercourse on days with optimal mucus secretions.

Thirdly, the use of an effective method for conception facilitates pregnancy occuring under optimal environmental conditions. Many factors, such as alcohol, smoking and caffeine consumption, body mass index outside the ideal range of 19–30, the use of medication or contact with potentially toxic products, are known to create detrimental environmental conditions for conception. Other precautions such as folic acid supplements at the time of conception can prevent birth defects. Efficient conception, similarly as efficient contraception, facilitates planned parenthood and therefore the care for the quality of reproduction.

Fourthly, the use of fertility awareness methods allows for the early detection of subfertility. Depending on the age as well as other factors, women with apparent delayed conception should be investigated at an early stage, using non-invasive techniques. Analysis of the basic fertility signs will yield important information on reproductive function, including the quality of the cervical mucus, the occurrence of ovulation and duration of the luteal phase. When obtained over a period of six months of attempting pregnancy, this information is a solid basis to decide on further management.

Finally, the comprehensive fertility awareness methods may help to avoid over-treatment as well as under-treatment of couples that desire pregnancy. Interventional treatments, such as IVF and ICSI, are increasingly used when a delay in conception exceeds one or two years without prior infertility investigations. Some of these couples are fertile but unawareness of the fertility period results in conception delay. It is well known that up to 25% of women on the IVF or ICSI waiting list conceive prior to treatment. With the increasing availability of assistant reproductive technologies, such as IVF and ICSI, there is a real risk that fertile but uninformed couples are treated unnecessarily.

3. Gametes, ovulation and fertilization

Male and female gametes are not equivalent

"I expose to men the origin of their first, and perhaps second, reason for existing." Leonardo da Vinci (1452–1519) wrote these words in around 1493 above his drawing *The Copulation* (fig 3.1). The Renaissance sketch shows a transparent view of the anatomy of sexual intercourse as envisaged by the anatomists of his time. The semen was supposed to come down from the brain through a channel, which can be seen in the spine of the man. In the woman the right lactiferous duct is depicted as originating in the right female breast and ending in the genital area. Even a genius like Leonardo da Vinci distorted his depictions of the bodies of man and woman to fit the ideology of his time and the notions of his commissioners, to whom he paid tribute. With this introduction, researchers at the Groningen university published, in 1999, magnetic resonance images of the male

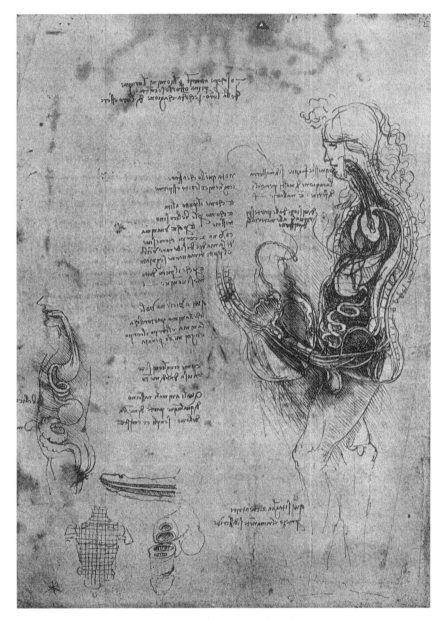

Figure 3.1 *The Copulation* as imagined and drawn by Leonardo da Vinci. Clark K, Pedretti C. *The drawings of Leonardo da Vinci in the collection of Her Majesty the Queen at Windsor Castle.* London: Phaidon, 1968.

and female genitals during intercourse, contributing to ow understanding of the exact anatomy, and correcting the anatomy of sexual intercourse as depicted by Leonardo da Vinci.

Today, in the discussion of gametes and fertilization, the spermatozoa and the egg are frequently considered equals in reproduction. Each of them provides half of the chromosomes for the formation of a new individual. However, the question can be raised whether they are biologically equal or not.

Sperms and eggs are strikingly different gametes. The reserve of eggs in humans is limited. Approximately four hundred eggs will mature during the reproductive life span. The production of sperms is continuous and it is estimated that the production during the life of a man amounts to some three thousand billion sperms. When the egg is released at the time of ovulation this cell is biologically almost as old as the woman, while the sperms at the time of release are not older than 70–80 days.

Also, genetically the eggs and sperms are not equal. Mature eggs before fertilization contain a larger amount of DNA than can be expected for a haploid cell. A significant amount of this DNA exists in the mitochondria. This amount increases by an active transcription process during the maturation of the egg. During the final maturation of the egg after the LH peak most of this DNA disappears, but a significant amount still remains. The question is: why do eggs contain such a large amount of mitochondria, when little is needed for their own existence? It can be speculated that the organelles are used during the early embryonic development. The mitochondrial DNA may contain the genetic information for the replication of the mitochondria and the synthesis of specific mitochondrial proteins and enzymes, which are required for the mitochondrial respiratory function. The amount of paternal mitochondria, which enter the egg at the time of sperm infiltration, may vary between species and today may also vary in the human when intracytoplasmatic sperm injection (ICSI) is used. However, the amount of maternal mitochondria largely dominates the paternal mitochondria by its sheer difference in volume.

Before ovulation the ovary receives a signal by the LH. During the period between this signal and fertilization the egg undergoes final maturation comprising an inductive phase of approximately six hours that is followed by a synthetic phase of approximately twelve hours. During this phase exchanges occur between the egg and the surrounding maternal cells in the follicle. Already, before fertilization, intensive contacts are made between the mother and the egg that is selected for ovulation and fertilization.

It can be argued that already at this stage the first individualization process of the potential embryo has been initiated. In any case, during this phase the mature egg is substantially different from the other eggs, which cannot be said for the sperms heading for fertilization.

Ovulation

The process of ovulation and ovum retrieval by the fimbriae was directly observed in humans for the first time at the Leuven Institute for Fertility and Embryology on May 2 1998 at 6.30 pm. It was a most intense moment to watch the release of the cumulus mass with the ovum from the ovary and the retrieval by the tubal fimbriae (fig 3.2).

The process was described in the scientific journal *Human Reproduction* in 1998 as follows: "The fimbriae on the ovulatory side appeared congested and tumescent and showed pulsatile movements synchronous with the heartbeat (of the woman). The cumulus mass was adherent to the fimbriae and released from the site of rupture by the sweeping movements of the fimbriae until it disappeared between the rigid fimbrial folds." The congestion of a rich vascular network in the fimbriae caused apparently sweeping movements in

Ovum capture in humans

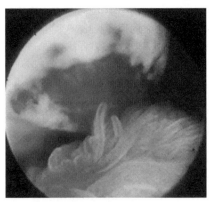 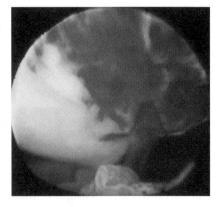

Figure 3.2 The cumulus oophorus containing the egg is stretched between the rupture follicle (top) and the tip of the fimbriae (bottom).

synchrony with the maternal heartbeat, while the cumulus mass with the egg was being transported into the Fallopian tube.

Fertilization

Fertilization occurs in the ampulla or the distal part of the Fallopian tube. This segment of the Fallopian tube has a complex system of mucosal folds covered by numerous ciliated cells. All these cilia are sweeping in the direction of the uterus and it is likely that sperms are also slowed down in their progression in this segment of the Fallopian tube. This would facilitate the process of fertilization.

The DNA synthesis of the embryonic genome starts after the penetration of the sperm into the egg and the formation of the pronucleus. The expression of specific embryonic (partially paternal) genetic material starts only after some cell divisions and becomes significant between the two-cell and eight-cell stages. During the first phase of the cell divisions the biochemical characteristics of a new individual are still absent, which implies that the first division and the mechanism of the first synthetic processes is quasi-exclusively controlled by the maternal genome and most likely via the enormous quantity of DNA present in the egg.

The sperm penetration is basically the signal to set off the developmental machinery in the mature egg. The time that the sperms were supposed to carry the "homunculus" are gone, but today the sperms also seem to lose their biological equality with the egg. The egg has a central role in the continuous cycle of life. It is no surprise that new life can be created without the input of sperms.

In 1972, Pierre Soupart, a Belgian scientist working as a Faculty member at the School of Medicine of Vanderbilt University in the US, obtained the first unquestionable evidence that the human egg could be fertilized in vitro. He applied to the National Institute of Health seeking support for extending in vitro fertilization experiments to their logical end by transferring the product of conception to a foster uterus. However, his application, which was approved for scientific merit with "high priority", was never activated due to the moratorium imposed by the Federal Government on any research in this area. In 1978, he succeeded in homogametic activation of the oocytes for the first time by inducing in vitro fusion of mouse oocytes followed by development of the product of conception to the blastocyst stage.

4. Implantation and placentation

Our knowledge of what happens between fertilization, when the fertilized egg is in the Fallopian tube, and the entering of the uterine cavity for implantation remains very scanty. There is apparently an intensive molecular crosstalk between the fertilized egg and maternal microenvironment in the tube and uterine cavity before implantation, which we unfortunately do not understand. Many embryos are lost during this period. The transport of the fertilized egg to the site of implantation is apparently tricky and dangerous in the development of a human being.

Implantation

In humans the uterus starts its preparation for implantation and pregnancy by a series of changes at the time of ovulation, which are called decidualization. The decidual reaction is initially under tight hormonal control by the mother allowing for a close interplay with the implantation of the blastocyst.

Implantation in humans is a complex process that is temporally and spatially restricted. It is a relatively short period of time, a matter of a few days, during the luteal phase of the menstrual cycle in which an embryo is "allowed" to successfully adhere to, and implant, within the uterus. Over the past decade, several genes and gene products that may participate in this process have been identified in the secretory phase endometrium.

The blastocyst is composed of outer cells, which develop into the trophoblast and later the placenta, and the inner cell mass. The trophoblast cells first attach the blastocyst to the uterine surface and then they penetrate the uterine epithelium and further invade the decidualizing tissue of the uterus at the site of implantation (fig 4.1). The surrounding maternal vessels are opened and colonized by the trophoblast. At the same time, the trophoblast produces hormones, such as the human chorionic hormone (hCG), to stimulate the production of steroid hormones by the ovary, which are necessary to maintain the decidualization of the uterine microenvironment.

Abnormal implantation can occur outside the uterus during transport through the Fallopian tube, which is not designed to support the placentation process. Placentation in the Fallopian tube leads to a

Deep placentation

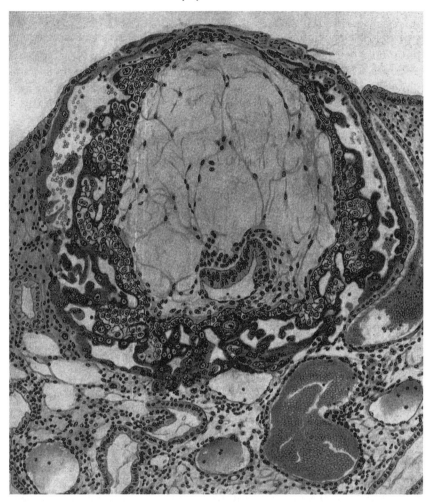

Figure 4.1 A drawing through the middle of an implantation site at the eleventh–twelfth day of development. The blastocystic trophoblast surrounds the blastocystic cavity. The endometrium is surrounding the conceptus (from Boyd & Hamilton, The Placenta, Heffer, 1970).

rupture of the tubal wall and is a life-threatening condition because of the uncontrolled intra-abdominal bleeding. The risk of a tubal pregnancy is increased whenever a sexually transmitted disease causes lesions in the mucosal folds of the Fallopian tube.

Deep placentation

In humans, the formation of a functional placenta requires the invasion of the fetal trophoblast not only into the decidua and inner myometrium (interstitial invasion), but also into the spiral arteries (endovascular invasion) of the uterus. In early pregnancy, the invading endovascular trophoblast effectively blocks perfusion to the developing fetus. This plugging of the spiral arteries by the trophoblast is thought to be critical to protect the early conceptus from exposure to an excess of reactive oxygen species. Later in pregnancy, the invading endovascular trophoblast replaces temporarily the endothelial lining, and most of the musculo-elastic wall of the spiral arteries thereby creating a high-flow, low-resistance circulation devoid of maternal vasomotor control. The process of the "disappearance of the normal muscular and elastic structures of the arteries and their replacement by fibrinoid material in which trophoblast cells are embedded" was first described by us in 1967 and we coined the changes as the physiological transformation of the spiral arteries. There is a general agreement that spiral artery remodeling reduces maternal blood flow resistance and increases utero-placental perfusion to meet the requirements of the developing fetus.

In 1976, Elisabeth Ramsey, a great researcher in placentation, pointed out that in primate species the depth of trophoblast invasion in the placental bed is apparently related to the degree of decidualization, suggesting a critical role for this process in determining the depth of trophoblast invasion. However, emerging evidence suggests that this extensive cellular differentiation process is also critical for tissue hemostasis prior to and during, pregnancy and that it confers cellular resistance to oxidative stress and inflammatory cytokines. Furthermore, the decidual process, which is associated with an influx of uterine natural killer cells and macrophages, plays an integral role in ensuring immunotolerance towards the semi-allogeneic feto-placental unit whilst simultaneously protecting mother and fetus against pathogens.

Human placentation is hemochorial, which means that the deeply implanted placenta is bathing in a sea of maternal blood while a thin placental membrane keeps the fetal and maternal circulations separate. Fetal development is fully dependent on the remodeling of the small spiral arteries in the inner uterine wall into large sinusoidal vessels. Before pregnancy these arterioles provide a circulation of some milliliters per minute, but at the end of pregnancy they have to supply more than 500 ml of blood per minute to the placenta.

The part of the uterus underlying the placenta with the utero-placental arteries has been coined the placental bed. It is a battlefield, where the maternal tissue is invaded by trophoblastic cells with the goal of adapting the maternal vessels to the needs of the developing fetus.

CHAPTER II

REPRODUCTIVE ECOLOGY

Human reproductive ecology pertains to reproduction and how it is influenced by environmental cues. In this chapter we discuss the role of the uterine microenvironment, the impact of the life in the womb on future health during adult life, and the contemporary dilemma of reproduction and emancipation.

5. The uterine microenvironment

One of the main features of Western society is the improvement of medical care for pregnant women. Fewer children are born, but the pregnancy is better planned and the conditions for the birth of a healthy child are steadily improving. The medical care has changed together with this evolution. The midwife and obstetrician used to be the professionals who took care of the delivery. Today, improved pregnancy outcome is largely dependent on the quality of medical care throughout pregnancy.

A striking example is the prevention of pre-eclampsia, a potentially dangerous complication that can occur in the second half of pregnancy, during labor, or in the period immediately after delivery. Pre-eclampsia is characterized by hypertension, abnormal amounts of protein in the urine, and other systemic disturbances. This condition affects about 3% of women. Eclampsia is an end stage of the disease, characterized by generalized seizures that potentially can kill the mother, the baby or even both, although rarely so in the developed world. Pre-eclampsia can not be prevented. It is managed by screening apparently healthy pregnant women and by inducing delivery when necessary. It is one of the most common causes of premature delivery.

For a long time the main concern was to avoid the potentially fatal eclamptic convulsions. Later, with the improvement of neonatal care, early delivery saved not only mothers but also many babies.

Subsequently, the goal was to prevent pre-eclampsia and the risks of fetal distress by starting medical treatment during the second trimester of pregnancy before the onset of clinical symptoms. However, attempts to prevent pre-eclampsia by initiating drug therapy in mid-pregnancy have failed.

Recent studies of the maternal blood supply to the placenta have shown that women who will develop pre-eclampsia later in pregnancy already have signs of an impaired maternal blood supply to the placenta (utero-placental blood flow) in the first trimester of pregnancy. Pre-eclampsia may therefore be preventable only when treatment is initiated immediately after or even prior to conception. As is the case with diabetes or neural tube defects, pregnancy outcome in women at risk of pre-eclampsia may already be determined by the uterine microenvironment at the time of conception.

What is the uterine microenvironment?

After ovulation, progesterone induces in estrogen-primed endometrium the expression of a highly co-ordinated gene set that initially defines a limited period of uterine receptivity (implantation window) and subsequently controls decidualization of the spiral arteries and surrounding tissues. The cellular responses to progesterone are complex and regulated at many levels. Target cells express various complements of membrane and nuclear receptors, each capable of differentially responding to hormonal activation. Furthermore, progesterone signaling in the reproductive tract is invariably intertwined with other hormones, cytokine, or growth factor signaling. Emerging evidence suggests that many of these "subsidiary" transcription factors physically interact with the progesterone receptor, thereby modifying the genomic response to progesterone. A major advantage of this system is that a single hormonal signal (progesterone) can elicit a highly co-ordinated cascade of cellular responses. A major disadvantage, however, is that a variety of aberrant signals can potentially disrupt the formation of these specific progesterone-dependent transcriptional complexes necessary for normal endometrial differentiation.

What can be wrong with the uterine microenvironment?

There is now abundant evidence that in diseases like endometriosis aberrations occur in the uterine microenvironment. The endometrium as well as the underlying myometrium are characterized by impaired tissue responses to progesterone. This is characterized by attenuated expression of progesterone-dependent genes during the luteal phase of the cycle as well as impaired repression of other gene sets. The concept of a relative progesterone insensitivity of the eutopic endometrium has been demonstrated in conditions like endometriosis. The concept is supported by the observation that progesterone treatment of mice inoculated with human eutopic endometrium inhibits development of endometriotic lesions when derived from disease-free women but not from affected patients. The underlying mechanism of relative progesterone insensitivity in endometriosis is not well understood, although there is strong experimental data to suggest that inflammation and activation of pro-inflammatory transcription factors can interfere with the progesterone receptor function.

Oxidative stress is a component of any inflammatory reaction, including endometriosis and pre-eclampsia. This is manifested in the endometrium by the altered expression of enzymes which are involved in defense against oxidative stress. The analogy between endometriosis and arteriosclerosis has been emphasized since both diseases are characterized by oxidative stress, the presence of tissue macrophages that express scavenger receptors, increased levels of oxidized lipoproteins and the presence of inflammatory cytokines and growth factors. There is an association between trophoblast invasion and oxidative stress in pre-eclamptic patients. Macrophages are probably involved in both oxidative stress and inhibition of trophoblast invasion. Finally, antioxidant treatment in a group of patients with increased risk of pre-eclampsia showed a potential benefit in the prevention of pre-eclampsia, which may therefore overcome the negative effects of a poorly adapted uterine microenvironment.

Multiple studies of the placental bed in pre-eclampsia and fetal growth retardation have shown that two processes are involved in the remodeling of the spiral arteries: a maternal decidualization process and the invasion of the placental bed by the fetal trophoblast. The fact that decidualization starts before the trophoblast invasion led to the hypothesis that a defective trophoblast invasion may be preceded by a defective decidualization process. Therefore, a defective progesterone response and impaired decidualization process may already set the stage for a defective deep placentation during the cycle of conception and result in pregnancy complications.

Defective deep placentation

Defective deep placentation is characterized by the absence of physiological remodeling of the myometrial spiral arteries in the placental bed and was first described by us in 1972 in patients with pre-eclampsia. The abnormality is manifested by the persistence of the normal structure of the spiral artery in the underlying myometrium (fig 5.1). Examination of hysterectomy specimens with the placenta in situ obtained from patients with pre-eclampsia and associated fetal growth retardation demonstrated that physiological remodeling of the spiral arteries was limited to just a few vessels in the center of the placental bed. Furthermore, hypertensive vascular lesions, such as

Human placentation

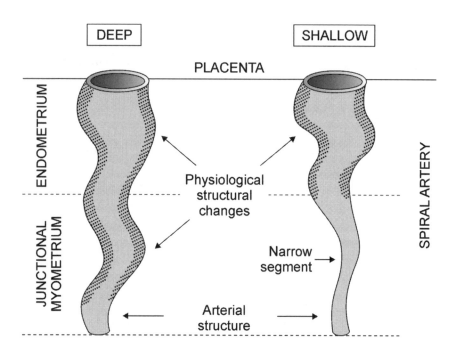

Figure 5.1 Utero-placental blood supply in normal (left) and abnormal (right) placentation.

thrombosis, acute atherosis and arteriosclerosis, were apparent in endometrial arterioles in and outside the placental bed. Variable degrees of defective physiological remodeling of the spiral arteries of the placental bed are found in a spectrum of complications of pregnancy, such as pre-eclampsia, placental abruption, preterm labor, preterm premature rupture of the membranes and fetal growth retardation.

Failure of the transformation of the spiral arteries in the placental bed is thought to increase the vascular resistance and to reduce the maternal blood flow to the placenta. However, it appears increasingly likely that additional factors, such as genetic predisposition (e.g. genetic thrombophilias), environmental factors (e.g. hormone disruptors) and pre-existing vascular pathology, modify the threshold for the clinical manifestations of defective deep placentation. Although pregnancy-induced hypertension and pre-eclampsia are likely to be multi-factorial disorders, there is strong clinical evidence to suggest that the degree of vascular resistance in the placental bed determines the feto-maternal outcome in these patients.

There is evidence to suggest that influences or manipulations of the uterine microenvironment can affect and improve implantation and deep placentation. In rodents, the decidual process can be triggered by local application of oil drops or tissue injury in the presence of elevated progesterone levels. In humans, random studies have shown an increased pregnancy rate in sub-fertile patients following hysterosalpingography with oil-soluble contrast medium. Conversely, suppression of inflammatory processes by GnRH-agonist therapy for three months has also been reported to improve IVF pregnancy in certain patients.

A major challenge in clinical practice is to refine our diagnostic tests so that medical intervention is not random but targets the underlying pathology. A case in point is the use of progesterone at the time of conception for the prevention of early pregnancy failure. Besides its direct effect on decidual transformation, progesterone has important local and systemic immuno-modulatory properties. The pharmacological use of progesterone during the luteal phase and in early pregnancy has fallen into disrepute, largely because it has been shown to be ineffective in the prevention of threatened sporadic miscarriage. However, in women with three or more consecutive miscarriages, in whom an underlying immunological cause is much more likely, progesterone treatment has been shown to significantly decrease the miscarriage rate compared to placebo or no treatment. Similarly, progesterone support improves pregnancy outcome after IVF treatment and two recent random trials have reported that progesterone also markedly reduced the incidence of preterm labor in at-risk patients.

There is strong evidence today that the quality of the uterine microenvironment during the cycle of conception is a major determinant of pregnancy outcome. Consequently, planning of pregnancy when the uterine microenvironment is optimal is highly important.

6. Life in the womb and future health

It is well known that environmental cues to which the pregnant patient is exposed during the first months of pregnancy can cause congenital anomalies. The teratogenic effects of some infections, chemicals, drugs, and irradiation during the early phase of pregnancy are well known. Furthermore, the increased use of recreational drugs, such as alcohol, cocaine and toluene (when sniffing glue) is another major risk factor of congenital abnormalities, often affecting those women who are already at increased risk of pregnancy complications because of poor social circumstances.

Fetal programming

During fetal growth and development the various organs and tissues of the body mature passing through varying 'critical periods' of rapid cell division. Changes in the nutrient and hormonal milieu at these times may alter the expression of the fetal genome, leading to permanent and irreversible effects on a range of physiological processes. The phenomenon of non-genetic transmission is termed fetal "programming". The hypothesis originated from studies of the death rates among babies born in Britain during the early 1900s. The geographical pattern of neonatal death rates was shown to closely resemble today's large variations in death rates from coronary heart disease. According to Barker's theory, the nutrient and hormonal milieu of the fetus alters gene expression, resulting in developmental adaptations that lead to permanent changes in physiology and metabolism, which in turn predispose to cardiovascular, metabolic and endocrine diseases in adult life.

Experimental studies in animals have documented many examples of fetal programming. Alterations in the mother's diet in pregnancy have, for example, been shown to program permanent changes in blood pressure, cholesterol metabolism, insulin secretion, and in a range of other metabolic, endocrine and immune parameters important in human disease. The obstetrical research group at the Catholic University in Leuven investigated how the altered glucose and aminoacid levels in the blood of the pregnant woman may affect the development of the baby. It has been known for many years that the newborn babies of diabetic mothers are less able to control their own blood sugar levels immediately after birth. Using experiments in rats they have shown that the abnormal maternal condition can affect the fetus and that abnormal circumstances such as diabetes and malnutrition badly affect not only the newborn baby, but also increase the risk for disease in adult life. The group compared the insulin-producing cells in the pancreas in the fetuses of normal, healthy pregnant rats with the pancreas of fetal rats whose mothers were diabetic. Pregnant rats can be made diabetic by giving the mother a single injection of a drug, streptozotocin. The results are aptly summarized by Peter Nathanielsz in his book *Life in the Womb: The Origin of Health and Disease*:

> A first generation of rats that were made diabetic at the beginning of pregnancy had high blood glucose levels throughout pregnancy. The high maternal blood glucose resulted in more glucose passing across the placenta to their fetuses, producing high fetal blood glucose. The elevated glucose in the fetal blood over-stimulated the fetal pancreas, and the cells that secrete insulin grew and divided at a greater than normal rate. When the challenge to the fetal pancreas was moderate, the pancreas enlarged, but did not collapse under the strain. When the maternal blood glucose was wildly out of control and as a result the fetal glucose was very high, the fetal ability to secrete insulin was exhausted under the excessive, unusual and constant challenge. The constant need to secrete more and more insulin to bring the very high blood glucose levels back to normal was eventually too much for the developing pancreas. It became exhausted by the effort to keep up with the large amount of glucose coming across the placenta from the diabetic mother.... Since the second-generation mothers have a decreased ability to secrete insulin, like their own mothers, they also will have a tendency to become diabetic when confronted with the challenge of pregnancy, exposing their own pups, the third generation, to high

levels of glucose during prenatal development. So it comes as no surprise that when these third-generation fetuses reached adulthood, they, too, demonstrated abnormal responses to a glucose tolerance test, having a decreased ability to secrete insulin in response to the glucose. Since the increased tendency of diabetes occurs in successive generations of pregnant mothers, there is no reason for it to stop passing across generations until maternal diabetes is controlled during pregnancy. When this is done, the fetal pancreas will not be excessively challenged during the development. That's the good news. Understanding how programming works will help us to prevent its adverse, unwanted effects.

Several recent studies have documented a causal link between low birth weight and chronic disease in adult life in humans. For instance, the evidence for an association between impaired fetal growth and increased risk of coronary heart disease is compelling. There are varying critical periods in fetal life during which organs and systems mature. Adverse intrauterine conditions during these different developmental stages are therefore likely to have specific short- and long-term consequences, leading to coronary heart disease, hypertension and diabetes during adult life.

These observations, linking impaired fetal growth with common adult diseases, point to a new developmental focus in disease prevention. However, it is premature to make policy recommendations, for example by introducing dietary supplements in an attempt to increase birth weight, as these interventions could in turn be harmful. Future long-term prospective studies should focus on collecting biological samples to increase our understanding of the underlying processes. As envisaged by Johan Eriksson, individual tailoring of lifestyle and pharmaceutical interventions according to early growth patterns and genetic setting may in the future maximize benefits in the prevention of cardiovascular disease and other diseases.

7. Reproduction and emancipation

Today's woman has her first menstrual period earlier in life and, although she has a longer reproductive life, she has fewer children and has them at a later age. The reliable and safe suppression of fertility has created opportunities for the modern woman that were unthinkable before. She can pursue uninterruptedly her professional aspirations, build a career and choose the appropriate time to have children. Clearly, however, the control of female fertility by contraception that has been achieved during the last fifty years has profoundly changed the reproductive pattern in certain societies. In Europe, the prediction of overpopulation made in the 1960s has now changed into a threat of underpopulation.

Are modern couples less fertile?

The lay press has paid much attention to studies reporting a decline in male fertility over recent decades. Although it remains to be established if semen quality is actually on the decline, the possibility of such a trend has raised concerns regarding the impact of environmental factors on human fertility. Apart from semen quality, the fertility of a couple is determined by numerous factors, many of which can change over time.

Recent studies measuring the time it takes to achieve pregnancy have produced conflicting findings. Fertility in Finland has reportedly decreased over recent decades, whereas in Britain and Sweden an opposite trend has been reported. It is likely that the increased fertility of couples, even in the face of decreased male fertility, is largely due to other factors, such as the eradication of diseases like gonorrhea or tuberculosis. However, changes in the availability of contraception and termination of pregnancy services make historical comparisons very difficult and it is probably impossible to identify the biological changes that have affected fertility over recent decades.

Women have increasingly fewer children. Although there is a highly significant correlation between the later age of the first child and the smaller size of the family, there is, however, no causal relationship. In other words, there is no evidence that the smaller size of families is a consequence of the delay in having children. Nevertheless, the postponement of the first pregnancy and the decrease in family size in Western Europe are matters of major concern.

Why do women want to stay childless?

In a recent valedictory address Edgar te Velde, an eminent fertility specialist at the University of Utrecht, discussed the woman's dilemma of reproduction and emancipation in modern society. It is estimated that 20% of girls born in 2002 will stay childless. Frequently it is assumed that they are unable to have children. Nothing is less true. The percentage of involuntarily childless women who will never be able to conceive remains limited to 2–4%. If the duration of involuntary infertility is set at 2–5 years, then the percentage as estimated by te Velde is 5–7%. Does this mean that the rest of the 20% is abandoning for some reason the wish to have children? The decision not to have children is apparently not a simple straightforward event but frequently involves a complex choice between career, lifestyle and motherhood. In our modern society women have full control of contraception, i.e. they decide when they do not want to become pregnant, but there is much less control of the timing of reproduction, i.e. when they want to become pregnant. The current control of fertility has largely been orientated towards the goal of contraception and much less to that of conception or achieving pregnancy.

The decision not to have children is in many cases not evident at all. Frequently, the decision has to be made at a time when career or modern lifestyle and motherhood are perceived to be in conflict. Women can make a choice, but if no decision is taken, the course of life will take over and decide whether or not they will have children. te Velde continued by describing how, when it is becoming too late, alternative options may still remain open. In the absence of the right partner, a woman may choose insemination with sperm from a donor with physical characteristics attractive to her. If her ovaries are depleted of eggs, she could purchase donor eggs as long as she has the financial means. A woman may not want to carry her baby throughout pregnancy or face the daunting delivery in which case she can pay for the services of a gestational carrier and receive her baby after birth.

While these options may be available to some, they are clearly not the solution for the current population problem. Moreover, the problem has given rise to the increased commercialization of human reproduction. It is no longer accepted as either normal or natural to have to wait for years to be become pregnant. With money, a woman can extend her reproductive life beyond the natural boundaries. She only has to pay royally for the magical services of the gynecologist who will make the impossible possible. The disturbing question is whether the commercialization of reproduction reflects an underlying attitude that pregnancy, including the baby, is a disposable and replaceable commodity in the modern world. Will time and money be the ultimate driving forces that control reproduction in the future?

CHAPTER III

INFERTILITY

Infertility exposes couples to a series of stressful conditions. Firstly, they are faced with the uncertainty of whether or not they are fertile; secondly, to know the cause of infertility they have to go through a period of investigation that may be long and, particularly for the woman, invasive; thirdly, in the event of achieving a pregnancy, infertile women have an increased risk of pregnancy complications; and finally, also more frequent for the woman than the man, they are faced with challenging treatments of uncertain outcome.

8. Who is infertile?

"Infertile" and "infertility" are confusing terms, which create, not infrequently, misunderstanding between physicians and patients. While fertility technology has made great progress in recent decennia the terminology has remained problematic.

Years ago, before ultrasound and sonography changed medicine, a teenager was referred to our gynecologic clinic for an ovarian cyst. She came with her mother. There was no cyst, but an advanced pregnancy. Heartbeats could be heard by listening with the Leffscope. The history of the girl revealed that she had irregular cycles and had had previous surgery for appendicitis. According to the mother the surgeon had told her that the daughter had polycystic ovaries and that she had no ovulations and was infertile. The mother could not believe that her daughter was pregnant as the surgeon had told her that she could not have children and, moreover, she said, her daughter was living at home and never went out. We had to take an X-ray to convince mother and daughter that they should be prepared for a delivery. Today, ultrasound has changed the diagnosis, but the understanding of polycystic ovaries and infertility still remains problematic.

In common language infertile and infertility mean "not fertile" and are equivalent to "impossible to conceive", or "not able to have a child" in the sense of sterile. Fertility is actual production of live off-spring and is the antonym of infertility. These definitions suggest that there is a dichotomy between fertility and infertility without grada-tion. A problem causing much confusion is that this descriptive def-inition of infertile has absorbed the "impossible to conceive" conno-tation from common parlance. Consequently, many patients and even clinicians tacitly assume, for example, that after one year of infertility the probability of conception is close to zero, which would justify immediate treatment.

In medical practice the terms infertile and infertility are used in a descriptive manner to indicate the duration of the delay in concep-tion after starting regular unprotected intercourse.

The most important question to be answered is when treatment is warranted or whether the couple should be encouraged to wait and try for a spontaneous pregnancy. Therefore, the prognostic statement is currently restricted to the chance of conceiving spontaneously within the following year. Such a chance is estimated to vary from a normal chance of at least 60% to 0% or sterility. In modern society age, previous use of contraception and a history of pelvic inflamma-tory disease or tubal pregnancy are important factors for estimating the prognosis.

Age

The association between male and female age and fertility is obscured by variables such as changes in sexual behavior with age and the ten-dency for sexual partners to be of similar age. In a French study of women having artificial insemination, because of male factor infertil-ity, the inseminations were timed to coincide with ovulation, thus con-trolling for intercourse behavior. That study provided convincing evi-dence of a biological decline in female fertility. By carefully controlling for the age of the woman and the variation in sexual behavior, some investigators found recently that the day-specific probability of preg-nancy declined with age for women from the late 20s onwards, with the probability of pregnancy twice as high for women aged 19–26 compared with women aged 35–39. From this study it can be con-cluded that women's fertility begins to decline in the late twenties with substantial decrease by the late thirties (Fig 8.1).

Conception and age

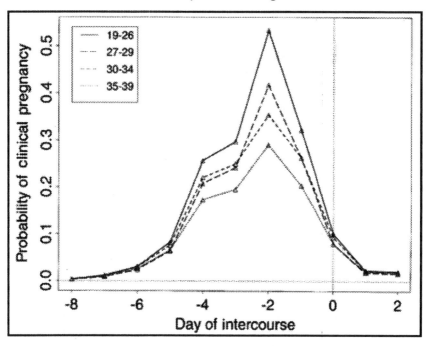

Figure 8.1. Probability of clinical pregnancy following intercourse on a given day relative to ovulation for women of average fertility aged 19–26, 27–29, 30–34 and 35–39 years. After Dunson et al. 2002.

Infertile women are also informed that the chance of a live birth following IVF treatment decreases with age. The chance of a live birth after IVF is significantly decreased after the age of 35 and is less than 10% after the age of 40 (Fig 8.2). On the other hand, after surgical treatment, as shown in cases of reversal of tubal sterilization, the chances of pregnancy are still surprisingly good in women over 40 years of age. In fact, the reported pregnancy rate after reversal of sterilization in patients aged ≥ 40 years ranges from 24–71%.

No comparable data are available regarding male infertility. Changes in semen characteristics with age have been studied and the preponderance of data suggest lower semen quality among men aged over 50 compared with men under 50. Fertility in men is less affected by age, but controlling for the age of the woman, fertility shows a significant decline by the late 30s.

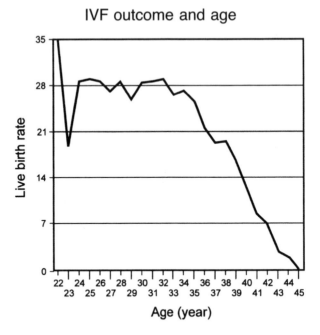

Figure 8.2. Age distribution and live birth rate among UK women receiving in vitro fertilization treatment between 1 April 2002 and 31 March 2003. Data from H.F.E.A. UK.

Contraception

It is likely that in a population with a high prevalence of modern contraception the time to pregnancy is prolonged. Previous use of hormonal contraception results in a modest but significant increase of the time to pregnancy that is dependent on the duration of use. The negative effect of previous combined oral contraceptive use on subsequent fertility is probably due to transient persistence of ovarian suppression or anovulation, particularly in susceptible women who had previously irregular cycles.

A large, German prospective study investigated women using natural family planning to find out whether the first cycle after stopping oral contraceptive intake had a normal duration. The mean cycle duration was significantly longer in the post-pill group up to the ninth cycle after pill discontinuation. However, a smaller Dutch study found that the first cycle after oral contraceptive discontinuation had a normal length. An explanation for the difference between both studies could be that in the Dutch study the mean age of oral contraceptive users was significantly lower than in the German study and, therefore, could have included women with a shorter duration of oral contraceptive use.

Long-term users of oral contraceptives are also likely to have less experience in fertility awareness methods, such as the vulvar mucus changes, to identify the days of fertility when they stop the pill and attempt pregnancy. They may also have less awareness of other subtle biological factors that promote intercourse during a woman's fertile days.

The use of an intrauterine contraceptive device (IUCD) has also been reported to be associated with conception delay. After short-term use the delay may be explained by the events for which IUCD use was prematurely discontinued, while long-term use in women who have never delivered a child appears to be associated with an increased risk of fertility impairment.

Pelvic inflammatory disease (PID)

Aside from AIDS, the most common and serious complication of sexually transmitted diseases (STDs) among women is pelvic inflammatory disease (PID), an infection of the upper genital tract. PID can affect the uterus, ovaries, Fallopian tubes, or other related structures.

Women with STDs – especially chlamydial infection and gonorrhea – are at greater risk of developing PID; a prior episode of PID increases the risk of another episode. Sexually active teenagers are more likely to develop PID than are older women. The more sexual partners a woman has, the greater her risk of developing PID.

Infertility occurs in approximately 20% of women who have had PID. The risk of infertility rises sharply with recurrent PID. Moreover, a woman who has had PID has a six-to-tenfold increased risk of tubal pregnancy. In the Fallopian tube the fertilized egg cannot implant normally and the ectopic placentation is life-threatening to the mother, and almost always fatal to her fetus. It is the leading cause of pregnancy-related death in developing countries and in African-American women. When a tubal pregnancy occurs during a first pregnancy there is also a 50% risk that the woman will not be able to conceive spontaneously again.

Early pregnancy loss

A recent Chinese population study on the time to pregnancy included, in addition to clinical pregnancy, the conception rate and early pregnancy loss. The overall per cycle conception rate was 40% over the first 12 months. The rate of clinical pregnancy was 30%. Approximately one-third of all the conceptions detected by urinary hCG failed to survive to delivery. More than two-thirds of these losses occurred before the pregnancy had been clinically recognized. The data are in agreement with other previous studies on early loss of pregnancy. The authors found no negative correlation between the early pregnancy loss and the time to clinical pregnancy, which led to the conclusion that early pregnancy loss can be regarded as a positive indicator that the stages of reproduction leading to implantation are intact.

With age there is an increased risk of miscarriage. The increased risk is likely to be related to the aging of the ovary and the higher risk of chromosomal abnormalities of the embryo. Some investigators suggest that clinical miscarriages are the result of a defective fetal-maternal signaling system, which causes a delay in the elimination of defective embryos.

9. The burden of investigations

The investigation of infertility in a couple involves a sperm analysis for the male and the exploration of the reproductive system including ovulation and normality of the Fallopian tubes and uterine cavity for the female. Such fertility investigation is complex and spread over time. The duration varies from a minimum of three months to one or two years. For the couple, fertility investigations are stressful and demanding, but, as the following example shows, the motivation of the couple for collaboration seldom has a limit.

A young Turkish couple was referred to the clinic and we explained that we wanted to know whether she had fertile cycles with ovulation and that his sperm was normal. She was asked to take her basal body temperature every morning for a period of six weeks and on return to bring a sperm sample for examination. When the couple came to the clinic six weeks later, she showed the chart with her daily temperatures and her husband proudly put a large bottle on the table, which contained his daily collections of sperm.

Full fertility investigation for the woman is invasive and expensive. Therefore, investigations are frequently delayed and spread over time. The delay may create insecurity and frustration for the couple, but it is based on the assumption that the longer the interval between the onset of attempts to become pregnant and the investigation or the longer the duration of infertility the lower the probability of a spontaneous conception.

The optimal approach in the management of female infertility requires that the timing and methods of the investigation be of benefit to the couple. The timing has important consequences for the couple. An early timing, when there is still a reasonable chance that pregnancy could occur spontaneously, may lead to unnecessary investigations and create a risk of overtreatment. A late timing may delay the diagnosis of a disorder for which an appropriate treatment exists, and unnecessarily prolong the burden for the couple. Treatments are also frequently attempted before the exploration is completed. Therefore, a delay in exploration of infertility may paradoxically favor overtreatment as well as undertreatment.

Early timing

It is currently recommended that people who have not conceived after one year of regular unprotected sexual intercourse should be offered an elementary clinical investigation including semen analysis and assessment of ovulation. It had been estimated, on the basis of earlier studies, that about 84% of couples will conceive within one year and 92% will do so within two years as long as they have regular sexual intercourse and do not use contraception. This represented an average monthly fecundity, defined as the ability to become pregnant in one month, of only 20%. However, human beings are apparently more fertile than is generally appreciated. Recently, two prospective studies have produced more optimistic figures. In a Chinese cohort study, the overall per cycle fecundability of couples wishing to conceive was 40% in the first 12 months. A European study found that 81% of women who practiced the "fertility awareness method" became pregnant within six months. This method is based on monitoring daily changes in vulvar mucus to identify the fertility window and peak fertility day in the cycle. By using the "fertility awareness method" unnecessary delays in conception can be avoided.

Using the fertility awareness method based on vulvar observations of cervical mucus, more than 80% of women will become pregnant within six months. Of the remaining 20%, approximately half will conceive spontaneously in the subsequent six cycles, resulting in 90% pregnancy rate in one year. Roughly half of the remaining 10% of unsuccessful couples can expect to conceive spontaneously in the next 36 cycles. After 48 unsuccessful cycles, the remaining 5% of couples should be considered sterile and spontaneous conception in this group is rare (Fig 9.1).

Time	Prevalence	Chance to conceive spontaneously in the future
After 6 unsuccessful cycles	About 20% at least slightly subfertile	50% of these couples likely to conceive in the next 6 cycles
After 12 unsuccessful cycles	About 10% at least moderately or seriously subfertile	50% of these couples will conceive spontaneously in the next 36 months
After 48 months	About 5% nearly completely infertile	Couples with only sporadic spontaneous conceptions

Figure 9.1. Definition and prevalence of subfertility and infertility in women using fertility awareness methods based on vulvar observations of cervical mucus. After Gnoth 2005.

Women who are able to use the vulvar mucus observations to determine the fertile days and peak day for timing the optimal days of intercourse and are not pregnant within three to six months can be informed that the monthly fecundibility is falling rapidly. In such patients it seems justifiable to offer an elementary fertility evaluation by a comprehensive fertility awareness method and sperma analysis.

Where there is a history of predisposing factors (such as amenorrhea, oligomenorrhea, pelvic inflammatory disease, low coital frequency or undescended testes), or factors which affect the fecundity in a normal population such as age over 35, early investigation should be offered. Where there is a known reason for infertility (such as prior pelvic surgery), early specialist referral should be offered.

Comprehensive fertility awareness method

The comprehensive fertility awareness method includes the daily recording of basal body temperature with indication of the days with vaginal bleeding, vulvar humidity and sexual intercourse. Analysis of these parameters over a period of three menstrual cycles will yield the basic information that is needed to determine the duration of the fertility window, the peak day of fertility, the presence of ovulation, the interval between ovulation and menstruation (i.e. the luteal phase of the cycle) and the frequency and timing of sexual intercourse.

The following advice can be given to women with regular cycles.
- During the *first three months* use vulvar mucus changes to time intercourse on the days of transparent, stretchy and slippery mucus observation. If no vulvar mucus changes can be observed during the menstrual cycle, ask for qualified advice on fertility awareness methods.
- During *the next three months* use the comprehensive fertility aware-ness method (including basal body temperature and sexual inter-course recordings) and attempt to time sexual intercourse on the peak mucus day. If no pregnancy occurs within the six cycles there is a 50% probability of a fertility problem.

Why is measuring basal body temperature useful?

A major aim of infertility investigations is to establish whether or not ovulation occurs regularly. Between the ages of 20 and 40 most women have regular ovulatory menstrual cycles. However, some women may not ovulate despite regular menstruations. Charting the changes in daily basal body temperature was historically the first test to determine if ovulation has occurred. After ovulation, the body temperature rises from 0.5 to 1°C and this hyperthermic plateau is maintained until the onset of menstruation. Today, tests for ovulation are usually done during the second part of the cycle and involve either measuring the blood progesterone levels or an endometrial biopsy. The histological dating was claimed to have the advantage of reflecting the cumulative effect of progesterone on the endometrium following ovulation and, hence, to provide more information on the "quality" of the luteal phase. However, to interpret the effect of progesterone on the endometrium, the timing of ovulation also needs to be determined, which is usually done by measuring the LH concentrations on daily urine or blood samples in order to detect the LH peak. The day of LH peak is then taken as the day of ovulation.

Recently, a large multi-centric study confirmed what many fertility specialists already suspected, namely that histological dating of endometrial biopsy timed by the urinary LH has no value for screening the quality of the luteal phase in patients with infertility. In addition, the investigators found that the urinary LH peak was a false sign of ovulation in more than 7% of women with or without infertility. In other patients there may be a delay in the onset of the luteal phase after the LH peak.

Since the endometrium biopsy is not providing the expected information on the quality of the luteal phase, plasma progesterone measurements is the preferred laboratory tool to determine the occurrence of ovulation and to assess the quality of the luteal phase. Unless progesterone levels are determined on daily samples there is no information on the onset of progesterone rise and, hence, the duration of the luteal phase. In the absence of a simple clinical tool, valuable information can be obtained by simply measuring the basal body temperature.

A one-stop investigation

The challenge in the investigation of female infertility is to make the investigation of the reproductive tract less invasive and less expensive. Currently, the hysterosalpingography (HSG) and laparoscopy are used for a complete investigation of the female reproductive tract.

The HSG is used to visualize the uterine cavity and test the patency of the Fallopian tubes. However, the technique is not without pain and risks. Apart from the exposure to radiation the main risk is infection, which occurs in 3% to 10% of patients depending on the presence of pelvic inflammatory disease. The procedure causes discomfort or even pain. Uterine cramping may result in a 17% false diagnosis of a bilateral tubal block.

Laparoscopy is used for the exploration of the tubo-ovarian structures and particularly the diagnosis of endometriosis and pelvic inflammatory disease. Laparoscopy is performed under general anesthesia and requires hospitalization. As laparoscopy is an invasive procedure, the diagnostic procedure is often combined with surgical treatment. Although this combined approach may be justifiable, it does not conform with the standard stratification for a surgical procedure that proceeds from diagnosis, to assessment of therapeutic options and, finally, operative interventions with informed patient consent.

Transvaginal hydrolaparoscopy has been recently introduced as a new diagnostic endoscopic technique that can be performed in the office or as an outpatient procedure. The patient lies in the dorsal position and, in contrast with laparoscopy, saline is used as a distension medium (Fig 9.2). The technique has the advantages that it provides direct access

Transvaginal hydrolaparoscopy

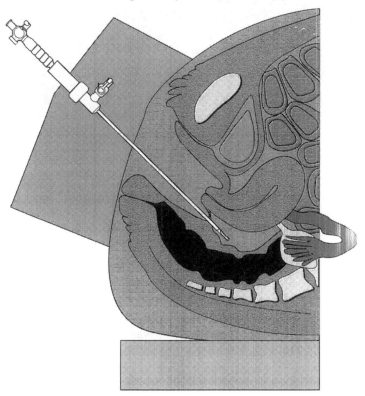

Figure 9.2. The access through the posteror fornix of the vagina gives direct access to the tubo-ovarian structures and with the small diameter needle-scope the organs are inspected under hydroflotation in their normal position without manipulation.

Transvaginal hydrolaparoscopy

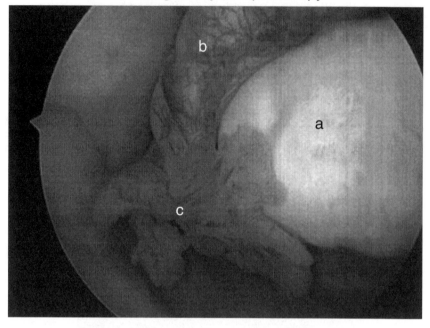

Figure 9.3. View under water during transvaginal hydrolaparoscopy of the ovary (a), Fallopian tube (b) and fimbriae (c).

to the tubo-ovarian structures and allows inspection of the organs under hydroflotation in their natural position without manipulation.

Transvaginal endoscopy combines both hysteroscopy and trans-vaginal hydrolaparoscopy as an office procedure and provides the information that is otherwise obtained by hysterosalpingography and laparoscopy (Fig 9.3). The major benefits of transvaginal endoscopy are that it is an office procedure, allows examination of tubo-ovarian structures and tubal patency. Accurate diagnosis can be made before surgery is proposed and discussed with the patient. The technique of transvaginal laparoscopy was developed at the Leuven Institute for Fertility and Embryology in 1997.

10. Increased risk of pregnancy complications

The increased incidence of feto-maternal complications in infertile patients is usually attributed to certain patient characteristics, such as older age or first pregnancy, or to the higher incidence of multiple pregnancies after fertility treatment. While this may be so, recent studies support the view that infertility is an independent risk factor for poor feto-maternal outcome. Perinatal mortality is increased in pregnancies conceived with the help of infertity treatment, but also for pregnancies among infertile couples not receiving treatment. Whether such pregnancy complications stem from the treatment or from the underlying disorder has been a long-standing question.

Which risks?

Several studies have reported that infertile couples are at increased risk of poor obstetrical outcome when compared with fertile couples. This association could not be explained by confounding factors such as multiple pregnancies, maternal age or parity. A recent large study found that singleton pregnancies in infertile women are also at increased risk of preterm delivery, fetal growth retardation and cesarean section, even if they are conceived without treatment. Several population studies have indicated that infertility treatment aimed at correcting the underlying factor is unlikely to be a major factor of adverse obstetrical outcome.

Infertility has also been associated with an increased risk of miscarriage although the available evidence is not very strong. A very recent large population-based study reported that a history of recurrent miscarriage, defined as two or more first trimester spontaneous losses, is associated with cervical incompetence, preterm premature rupture of membranes, and preterm labor, independent from the effects of other risk factors. This would suggest that certain pathological processes involved in infertility predispose for a spectrum of pregnancy complications such as spontaneous miscarriage, preterm delivery, pre-eclampsia and fetal growth retardation. These epidemiological studies provide support for the notion that a common etiology underpins infertility, early pregnancy failure and late obstetrical complications.

The lack of consensus in diagnostic criteria and the heterogeneous nature of contemporary infertility investigations make it very difficult to define the risk of adverse pregnancy outcome in relation to specific reproductive disorders, such as endometriosis, polycystic ovary syndrome, tubal inflammatory disease or other disorders. At least a quarter of all infertile couples have unexplained infertility. A recent study analyzed the obstetrical history and perinatal outcome of 498 couples with unexplained infertility, defined as having normal semen parameters, ovulatory cycles and patency of both Fallopian tubes. After adjusting for age, parity and multiple pregnancies, the authors found a significantly higher incidence of pre-eclampsia, placental abruption and preterm labour in women with unexplained infertility compared to the general obstetric population.

While infertility itself has been recognized as a risk factor for impaired pregnancy outcome, a recent study based on the Danish national birth cohort showed that a long time to pregnancy per se is a marker for increased risk of peri-natal mortality. Mothers waiting for longer than one year to conceive their first child gave birth to babies with a higher risk of neonatal death compared with children conceived sooner.

Aberrant uterine microenvironment

It has taken many years for fertility specialists to realize that successful treatment of infertility is not pregnancy but the birth of a single, healthy, term baby. The epidemiological evidence for a pathological link between infertility and poor feto-maternal outcome raises a number of important challenges and opportunities in clinical practice.

Firstly, the data emphasizes the importance of peri-conceptual care for the prevention of not only early pregnancy loss but also late obstetrical complications such as pre-eclampsia and preterm labor. Successful deep placentation depends on the remodeling of uterine tissues prior to, and from the early onset of, pregnancy. The corollary of this observation implies that medical intervention aimed at preventing late obstetrical complications is likely to be effective only if initiated during the peri-conceptual period.

Secondly, treatment should be targeted and much more effort should be placed on defining the biochemical perturbations in the uterine microenvironment prior to pregnancy.

New technologies, such as micro-array and proteomics, raise the possibility that diagnostic 'finger prints' will be discovered in endometrial or blood samples of women at risk for pregnancy complications. Micro-array technology allows simultaneous analysis of the expression of large numbers of genes. This technology has been

used to characterize the expression of genes, gene families and signal transduction pathways in the endometrium of women with
endometriosis. Recent data support the hypothesis that endometriosis is associated with dysfunction of specific gene sets, leading to an
inhospitable environment for implantation. Finally, there is an
urgent need for a national or international framework that co-ordi-
nates large, well-conducted, prospective, randomized trials assess-
ing the safety and effectiveness of peri-conceptual medical treatments.

11. The challenge of infertility treatment

Attempts to restore fertility have always been celebrated. However,
the laudable intention of assisting in creating new life may be the reason why reproductive medicine has paid so little attention to the
harm it may cause despite the ancient adagio "first, do not harm". In
fact, there are major pitfalls and risks of harm on the road to restore
fertility.

Pregnancy despite treatment

An old and major pitfall is that most couples with infertility are not
sterile, but experience a delay in conception. At any time a spontaneous pregnancy can occur, which is unrelated to the treatment.
However, it is tempting for both doctor and patient to draw the conclusion that the treatment was successful. Indeed, many treatments of
infertility have been based on the belief, but not the scientific proof,
that the pregnancy that occurred during or after treatment was treat-
ment-related. Obviously, unproven and useless treatments are a
waste of time, money and, not infrequently, a cause of more harm
than good.

A classic example of a harmful treatment was the use of the synthetic estrogen diethylstilbestrol (DES) for the treatment of miscarriage. The treatment was not only without benefit, but intrauterine
exposure to DES caused damage to the development of the genital
tract of the female fetus, creating a risk of developing a vaginal cancer in early adulthood. In addition, as shown recently, the exposure
during intrauterine life to DES is associated with increased risk of
uterine fibroids and endometriosis during reproductive life.

Although medical therapies are extensively investigated before they are introduced, there is no test to prove that there is no harm and doctors need to think about harm all the time.

The paradox of tubal surgery

With the advent of microsurgical techniques there was great hope that surgery could restore fertility in patients with blocked Fallopian tubes. PID is in most cases the cause of the blockage of the Fallopian tubes. In severe cases the infection causes, in addition to the blockage, extensive damage of the mucosal lining of the Fallopian tube. With the introduction of microsurgical techniques in the 1970s tubal patency could be restored in the majority of the cases, but the mucosa remained damaged. As a consequence, the pregnancy outcome in terms of a normal intrauterine pregnancy was a great failure. The majority of women did not get pregnant and, in the case of pregnancy, the implantation occurred more frequently in the Fallopian tube than in the uterus leading to the life-threatening condition of a tubal pregnancy. The poor results and increased risk of tubal pregnancy, particularly in patients with PID, were a cause of desperation for patients and surgeons.

Tubal infertility is at present a condition that illustrates the medical risks when IVF is not accepted or available as an alternative solution. Centers that offer surgery only for tubal sterility may expose the patient to an increased risk of tubal pregnancy. Centers that offer both reconstructive tubal surgery and IVF can offer the appropriate treatment depending on the severity of the disease. With proper selection a minority of patients will today be offered reconstructive surgery. In patients with established poor prognosis it is even advisable to remove the Fallopian tubes prior to IVF to increase the implantation rate and reduce the risk of tubal pregnancy.

The following case illustrates the complexity of tubal infertility.

Married in 1971 at the age of 22 Christiane, a teacher, took the pill for about one year. At her first gynecological examination a large cyst on the right ovary was found. The gynecologist decided to remove the right adnexa, which means the ovary (with the cyst) together with the Fallopian tube. The diagnosis was an ovarian endometriotic cyst. She was advised to take Orgametril for four months. In 1973 she consulted another gynecologist. A hysterosalpingography (HSG) was performed and showed that the distal end of the left Fallopian tube was obstructed. The young couple were hopeless: the right ovary and tube had been removed and the left tube was blocked. She consulted another gynecologist who wanted to see the HSG which could not be found. A new HSG was performed, which confirmed the distal obstruction of the left Fallopian tube. This was the history when she came to our university infertility clinic. The couple were in a very depressed state.

The couple had a full fertility investigation. Her previous history included an appendectomy at the age of 12. He had a negative history and the spermiogram was normal. Her basal body temperature was biphasic and an endometrium biopsy confirmed ovulatory cycles. The laparoscopy showed a 2 cm endometrioma on the left ovary and the distal end of the Fallopian tube was fixed and occluded by adhesions between the ovary and the pelvic wall. The tubal patency test confirmed distal obstruction of the tube without distension of the tube. It was explained to the couple that the chances for pregnancy were less than 1% and that the only possibility remaining was conservative surgery with ablation of the endometrioma and reconstruction of the ovary and the restoration of the Fallopian tube patency and mobility. There was no sign of pelvic inflammatory disease and we estimated that by using microsurgical techniques the chances of pregnancy could be as high as 60%.

The surgery was performed in May, 1975. During a three-hour microsurgical procedure the distal tubal end was mobilized and the patency fully restored. The mucosal lining of the ampullary segment was well preserved. She should have a good prognosis after all! The risk for a tubal pregnancy should also be low. Indeed, in October 1975, she became pregnant. However, at 13 weeks gestation she had slight bleeding, which was followed by a miscarriage.

She failed to conceive again and had a medical treatment to improve ovulation, but also without success. In December 1977, she had a control laparoscopy which showed that the distal end of the left tube was in relatively good condition with a slightly retracted opening. In 1978, she again received medical treatment for ovarian stimulation for several months without success. In 1979, adoption was proposed, and she also had a control HSG. The HSG confirmed the patency of the left tube, but also showed the presence of a uterine fibroid bulging into the uterine cavity. This was apparently a new visible pathology which was not seen on the previous HSGs. Surgery was proposed to remove the uterine fibroid. In april 1979, a 2 cm large submucus fibroid was removed. She conceived spontaneously soon after surgery and delivered a healthy boy by cesarean section in June 1980.

It took many years for this couple to achieve a successful pregnancy. Today, the story would be different, but not necessarily more successful. After the diagnosis of a hydrosalpinx the patient would have been referred for IVF. It is very likely that the remaining tube with the hydrosalpinx would have been removed in order to improve the chances of IVF. This would have eliminated the possibility of a spontaneous pregnancy, but whether or not she would have conceived with IVF remains very questionable as she had an undiagnosed uterine pathology.

Failure of tubal transplantation

During the last century transplantation has been one of the greatest medical successes. In 1954, a kidney was transplanted, for the first time, from one healthy identical twin to the other twin who was dying of renal disease at the Brigham Hospital in the US. The most spectacular transplant, however, was the first human heart transplant by Chris Bernard at the Groote Schuur Hospital, South Africa, in 1967. The first attempt to perform tubal transplantation in the human was also performed by gynecologists at the Groote Schuur hospital. The tubal transplantation, however, failed due to tissue rejection and ended dramatically with a life-threatening sepsis.

In the 1970s we investigated the possibility of tubal transplantation in rabbits by microsurgical techniques. While the transplant was technically a success it was not applied to women because of the risk of rejection which was estimated to be too high to justify attempts in humans. Moreover, a fear existed that the immune suppressive therapy given to prevent the rejection of the transplanted organ could be harmful for the fetus.

Sterility: the hard road to the truth

In most cases the diagnosis of sterility is not made and the road to the truth remains long and frustrating. After many years of anticipation and failed attempts the couple slowly come to realize that pregnancy will not occur and the age factor destroys any further hope. The loss of time and energy in such cases is frequently due to several factors. Firstly, the couple may have been waiting too long before seeking help. Important aspects of life, such as a career, expansion of a business or finding a home may have postponed the search for medical assistance. Secondly, the long road of fertility investigations, the absence of clear explanation and unsuccessful therapeutic trials may have caused much loss of time.

The confrontation with the problem of sterility is also very challenging for a fertility team. From the age-old attitude, which was to respond to sterility with adoption or foster parenthood, the team can respond in two ways. Firstly, the infertility investigations are organized and scheduled to arrive at a conclusion within a reasonable period of months, rather than years. Secondly, there should be a willingness to respond to the demands of the sterile couple and to consider other solutions for sterility, such as artificial insemination with donor sperms in case of male sterility and, when assisted reproductive technologies, such as in vitro fertilization, are available, they should not be rejected, but carefully considered. The evaluation of the medical, psycho-social and ethical aspects of artificial insemination and assisted reproductive technologies will be discussed in further chapters.

CHAPTER IV

RISKS OF IN VITRO FERTILIZATION

In this chapter we evaluate briefly the medical risks and the potential complications of the new assisted reproductive technologies (ART) for patients and their offspring. The first IVF baby was born in 1978. The technique of intracytoplasmatic sperm injection for the treatment of male infertility was introduced in 1992. Both these techniques were introduced with little knowledge of the risks at the time of introduction. Until recently, these techniques were considered appropriate substitutes for natural oocyte fertilization, and were therefore regarded as safe. However, reports of children conceived by ART and presenting health problems have been published in recent years. Assisted reproduction now accounts for 1–3% of births in developed countries. The safety and quality of reproduction in patients using these techniques needs to be closely monitored and evaluated. The quality of the laboratory procedures and the management in cases of IVF blunders also raise questions.

12. Complications during treatment

Medical

IVF treatment is not without risks for the patient's health and complications may occur at different stages. During the initial phase the hormonal stimulation of the ovaries results in an ovarian hyperstimulation syndrome (OHSS) in 3–7% of the patients. Although the complication is usually mild, in the severe form the patient suffers from pain and water retention with the risk of heart decompensation and renal damage. Despite many years of clinical experience the patient at risk cannot always be identified before treatment and there is no possibility to completely prevent severe OHSS, except by withholding the injection of the ovulation-trigger hCG. Individualization of treatment according to specific risk factors and the monitoring of the response during the treatment cycle with the option of freezing all embryos, or replacement of only a single embryo, have the potential to reduce the risk and the severity of the syndrome in susceptible cases. Mortality has been reported, but its incidence is unknown as there is no registration of mortality.

Egg aspiration can cause mild complications such as pain, bleeding or infection. Mild bleeding usually stops spontaneously. Heavy bleeding even with fatality and severe infection has been reported, but again there is no prospective registration to have an accurate estimation of the incidence.

Embryo transfer has also been reported to result in ectopic implantation, particularly in patients with tubal infertility. Even in cases where a Fallopian tube has been removed, the risk of a pregnancy in the intramyometrial segment of the Fallopian tube persists. Such an intramural pregnancy is a life-threatening complication.

Psychological

The psychological stress endured by a couple during treatment with assisted reproductive techniques should not be underestimated. Dropout is a well-known phenomenon in IVF-ICSI and is, in the majority of cases, related to psychological factors. The enormous stress and frustration increase during the course of treatment. A recent large German IVF study found that the dropout of non-pregnant patients increased from 40% after the first cycle to 62% after the fourth cycle. A Scandinavian study involving almost a thousand couples found that the majority of the couples (54%), which did not achieve a live birth, chose not to proceed through the fully subsidized treatment program consisting of three complete IVF cycles. The majority of these discontinuations were due to psychological stress.

During IVF treatment couples are is exposed to many ups and downs. Moreover, the treatment fails in about 50% of cases. It is not so much the treatment as the uncertainty of the outcome which is stressful for the couples. To reduce the stressful conditions, the University Medical Center St Radboud in The Netherlands has initiated a project that is an interactive digital infertility clinic. Couples participating in the project receive their personal results on sperm quality, ovarian stimulation, egg aspiration, fertilization, quality of embryos, together with proposed treatments and, at regular times, chats with the medical personnel at home via internet. The provision should enforce the patient's position. When better informed, they are better able to make their own decisions during the period of IVF treatment. The project intends to evaluate whether the interactive information system helps to improve the circumstances that allow couples to make their own decisions about whether or not they should continue with the treatment. The project underlines the importance of offering continuing support to an infertile couple by a dedicated team.

13. Multiple pregnancy

Hormone treatments for infertility have made multiple pregnancy a major clinical problem. The incidence of multiple pregnancy increased with the use of ovarian stimulating hormones for the treatment of infertile patients with ovulatory problems. However, the issue became a major problem when more and more patients with different causes of infertility were treated with IVF and received hormone stimulation. The risk of multiple pregnancy is the most obvious complication of in vitro fertilization and embryo transfer. After poor results in the early years of IVF it was found that the systematic transfer of more than one fertilized egg increased the chances of pregnancy, but this practice also increased the risk of multiple pregnancy. It is quite obvious that the risk of multiple pregnancy is largely related to the number of embryos transferred to the uterus. The strategy of transfering fewer embryos resulted in fewer multiple pregnancies. During the last decade the risk of multiple pregnancy has decreased in Belgium from 30–35% to 23–25%. The recent strategy of transfering only one or two embryos is likely to decrease the risk of multiple pregnancy to more normal levels.

The risks associated with a multiple pregnancy are well known. In a normal population, the relative risks of low birth weight and perinatal mortality in twin pregnancy are respectively 10 and 6 times higher than for singletons. An important consideration, however, is that there is a difference between the risks of twin pregnancy after IVF and spontaneous conception. A recent systematic review comparing the perinatal outcome of twin pregnancies between natural and assisted conception found that, for twin pregnancies after assisted conception, the perinatal mortality is about 40% lower than

after natural conception. Therefore, the complications of a twin pregnancy after IVF are not fully comparable with those of a twin pregnancy after spontaneous conception. There may be several reasons
for this discrepancy. The main reason is that a twin pregnancy after
in vitro fertilization is less likely to be monozygotic or monochorionic. A monochorionic twin gestation is, for example, a leading risk
factor for very low birth weight. This may to some extent explain the
paradoxical finding that after IVF and embryo transfer the risk of low
for gestational age birth weight is increased in singleton pregnancy,
but not in twin pregnancy.

Embryo reduction

The epidemic of multiple pregnancies has resulted in catastrophic
increases in morbidity and mortality, and in increased economic costs
to society. Multifetal pregnancy reduction has been used to reduce an
excessive number of fetuses in the late first trimester and has significantly improved outcome.

A recent report from 11 centers in 5 countries involving 3513 cases
concluded that multifetal pregnancy reduction outcomes improved
considerably with experience. Reductions from triplets to twins and
from quadruplets to twins carry outcomes as good as those of unre-
duced twin gestation. In terms of losses, prematurity, and growth,
higher starting numbers carry worse outcomes.

However, the procedure carries with it medical, ethical and psychological issues for both the parents and the physicians involved.
The emotional and psychological traumas experienced by the women
during the procedure are of great concern, even in social situations
where abortion is accepted. Each of the surviving children can claim
that their brother or sister was killed before he or she was born.

The terrible consequences of the complications of a partially failed
embryo reduction procedure can be appreciated from the following
case report presented at the annual meeting of the American Society
of Reproductive Medicine in 2002.

The patient, 29 years old, underwent ICSI-IVF after four failures in the
past. There were two implantation failures and two early pregnancy losses.
She formed eight embryos and since it was her fifth attempt, all were
replaced on day two. This resulted in a quintuplet pregnancy. It was decided

to reduce the fetuses to twin pregnancy at 8.5–9 weeks in view of her early pregnancy losses. Selective fetal reduction was carried out transvaginally under ultrasound control. Mechanical trauma to the heart was elected as the method of choice in view of previous poor experience of chorioamnionitis with intracardiac injection of potassiumchloride. Two fetuses were successfully reduced. The third elected sac was entered and the same procedure applied to this fetus. However, the heart could not be entered and fetal injuries were caused at other places. The needle was removed and a re-entry was tried. This resulted in the entry of a big vessel in the myometrium and a hematoma was seen in the myometrium. The procedure was abandoned and the whole situation was explained to the couple. They were informed that a second attempt was mandatory since the fetus had been reasonably traumatized. After the procedure the patient started bleeding and was treated conservatively. The hematoma resolved in four weeks, but there was also drainage of liquor from the affected sac and the fetal heartbeat slowed down to 70–80/minute. It was decided that the sac be left alone since fetal demise was imminent. However, rescanning 15 days later at 14 weeks showed reforming of liquor and the cardiac activity improved. Due to strong religious beliefs and superstitions, the couple refused further intervention. All possible consequences and risks were discussed with them and a written consent for no further intervention was taken. During pregnancy, the two normal fetuses showed normal growth, activity and normal liquor. The reduced fetus also showed normal growth, but movements were restricted and there was complete flexion of the spine. At 34 weeks an elective cesarean section was done for fetal distress. The reduced fetus, a female, was in good condition and did not require any resuscitation. The following malformations were noted: cleft lip and palate, extensive webbing of the neck due to contractures, absence of right lower jaw, kyphoscoliosis, bilateral talipes equino and contractures of the right elbow and right knee joint. Most of the malformations were due to the drainage of liquor, but the fetus had also been traumatized by the procedure.

To the knowledge of the author this was the first case report of a live baby being born after failed selective fetal reduction.

Single embryo transfer

The recent strategy of using the transfer of only one or two embryos is likely to significantly decrease the risk of multiple pregnancy, but might also result in considerable decline in the overall birth rate. In

1998, IVF centers in Belgium and Scandinavia started to identify patients suitable for single embryo transfer. The group at the University of Ghent published a paper in 1998 with the provocative title "Who's afraid of single embryo transfer?"

A recent review identified that, in the period 1995–2004, four randomized controlled trials and seven observational studies using fresh embryo transfers were published. The analysis of the randomized papers showed that in good prognosis patients satisfactory delivery rates can be achieved with elective single embryo transfer (SET). The delivery rate is, however, significantly lower after SET compared with double embryo transfer (DET). The lower delivery rate might be restored with the addition of frozen-thawed embryos in these patients. Elective SET defined as the transfer of one good embryo in cases where at least two good quality embryos are available, results in a dramatic decrease in multiple births. The results of the observational studies indicate that the pregnancy and delivery rates achieved with SET and DET are similar. The reason for achieving similar results is of course that the two groups are not strictly comparable: good prognosis women receive SET, while poor prognosis women receive DET. Should all patients have received DET, the overall pregnancy and delivery rates would have been higher but at the price of a higher multiple pregnancy rate.

A few health economic analyses have evaluated SET versus DET, including treatment costs, maternal delivery costs and neonatal costs. However, these studies are not based on a large population randomization between SET and DET. Nonetheless, cost analyses performed so far have been in favor of SET.

In Belgium, new legislation introduced in 2003 provides reimbursement for six cycles of IVF for women under 43 years of age provided that the following criteria are met:
- Aged 35 or younger: first cycle, single embryo transfer; second cycle, one or two embryos per transfer if there is no availability of good quality embryos; third to sixth cycle, maximum of two embryos per transfer;
- Aged 35–39 years: first and second cycle, maximum of two embryos transferred; third to sixth cycle, maximum of three embryos per transfer;
- Aged over 39: no maximum on number of embryos transferred;
- For thawed frozen embryos, two embryos maximum.

The first reports on the application of the law show a decrease in twin pregnancies from 20% to less than 5%. These results need to be confirmed and evaluated by larger studies. Since randomized, controlled trials show lower pregnancy and delivery rates after eSET compared to DET, one would have expected a decline in delivery rate. However, since no remarkable decline in delivery rates is notable, a better selection of embryos for transfer ought to have taken place and/or better prognosis women have been treated. The price, which has to be paid for the decrease in multiple birth rates, seems to be a slight decrease or the absence of an increase in the delivery rate. This means that women have to go through more cycles to achieve a live birth. The associated inconvenience and psychological stress should also be kept in mind. However, if these additional cycles can be restricted to some freezing-thawing cycles not requiring ovarian stimulation and oocyte aspiration this stress would be regarded as minor and must be balanced against the much higher risk of multiple pregnancy.

The introduction of six subsidized cycles in Belgium has already resulted in a very substantial increase in the number of IVF cycles. The question arises whether the subsidized access to an IVF center will result in a preferential use of IVF as a first choice treatment for infertility and will couples with fertility problems in the future be referred straightaway to assisted conception?

14. Child and adult health risks

Risks of birth defects

A recent review of all papers published by March 2003 provided interesting data relating to the prevalence of birth defects in infants conceived following IVF and/or ICSI compared to spontaneously conceived infants. Twenty-five studies were identified satisfying strict criteria, which were defined *a priori* to determine whether studies were suitable for inclusion in a meta-analysis. The results showed that two-thirds of the studies found a 25% or greater increased risk of birth defects in ART infants. The results of meta-analyses of the seven reviewer-selected studies and of all 25 studies suggested a statistically significant 30–40% increased risk of birth defects associated with ART. At present it can be concluded that all suitable published studies suggest that children born following IVF are at increased risk of birth defects compared with spontaneous conceptions. The authors concluded that this information should be made available to couples seeking ART treatment.

An excess of birth defects in IVF and ICSI infants is biologically plausible. Factors associated with ART treatment that may increase the risk of birth defects include the underlying cause of infertility in the couples seeking treatment, and factors associated with the IVF/ICSI procedures themselves such as medications, delayed fertilization of oocytes, the effects of culture and the freezing and thawing of embryos.

To which extent reproduction itself in the test-tube population may be affected has not yet been assessed. In the near future an increasing number of test-tube babies will be adults and will allow the evaluation of the reproductive potential of this population.

Low birth weight

Prospective and retrospective follow-up studies of children born as a result of assisted reproduction have shown that the development is normal and similar to the general population. Neonatal data, however, have indicated a lower birth weight in the IVF and ICSI singletons as compared with naturally conceived children. The major risk is the increase of babies with a low and very low birth weight for age. At 37 weeks or later the risk of low birth weight is 2.6 times higher than in a normal population.

A recent systematic review of controlled studies published between 1985 and 2002 found that singleton pregnancies from assisted reproduction have a significantly worse perinatal outcome than non-assisted singleton pregnancies. The risks after IVF and ICSI were more elevated for very preterm and preterm births, small for gestational age infants, cesarean section, admission to a neonatal intensive care unit and perinatal mortality.

Several articles published over recent years warn of the implication of assisted reproductive techniques on subsequent fetal growth, birth weight and adult health. A call has been made for long-term analysis of children conceived by ART, primarily because of the epidemiological link between small for gestational age babies and adult onset diseases, such as cardiovascular disease and type II diabetes or the fetal origins of adult disease such as was proposed in the hypothesis of

Barker. The unanswered important question is whether the reason for the low birth weight lies in the hormonal treatment, the manipulations and environment during the in vitro period or the underlying condition of infertility itself.

Epigenetic risks

Some reproductive techniques that have been developed are quite invasive such as ICSI using mature and immature sperm cells for fertilization, the biopsying of embryos for preimplantation genetic diagnosis (PGD) and transfer of ooplasm to a recipient oocyte. Apart from the risk of birth defects there is the unknown long-term risk that epigenetic reprogramming events in the gametes and early embryos may occur. In addition, a broader causal model linking environmental stressors with phenotype perturbation through both transcriptional and epigenetic modification of gene expression has been suggested.

Child health

A recent multi-center cohort study evaluated the physical health of 5-year-old children conceived after intracytoplasmic sperm injection, in vitro fertilization and a matched comparison group of naturally conceived children in five European countries. The detailed study of 1515 children showed that rates of major malformations were significantly higher in ICSI compared to the natural conception group and were little affected by adjustment for socio-demographic differences. IVF children had a similar pattern of increased congenital anomalies, but this did not reach statistical difference. The higher rate observed in the ICSI group was partially due to an excess of malformations in the urogenital system of boys. Bearing in mind that only children born after at least 32 weeks of gestation were included in the study, the ICSI/IVF children were nevertheless still a little less mature, a finding that is consistent with previous studies on birth weight. The ICSI and IVF children were more likely than naturally conceived children to have had a significant childhood illness, to have had a surgical operation, to require medical therapy and to be admitted to a hospital. The authors concluded that the findings were generally reassuring. However, the finding that ICSI children presented significantly more major congenital malformations and both ICSI and IVF children were more likely to need health care resources than naturally conceived children means that ongoing monitoring of these children is required.

In conclusion, assisted reproductive technologies now account for between 1% and 3% of annual births in many Western countries and the in vitro fertilization services are growing worldwide. Pooled results from all suitable published studies suggest that children born following ART are at a 25% or greater risk of birth defects compared to spontaneous conceptions. There is evidence of a significant increase in low birth weight and preterm delivery among singletons conceived with all types of ART; however, there remains uncertainty about whether these risks stem from the treatment or the parental infertility. There is inconclusive evidence that ART may be associated with genetic imprinting disorder.

In the presence of a significant increase in birth defects and low birth weight there is a need for continuing surveillance of the infant, including monitoring birth defects, development, reproduction and cancer. Larger, population-based studies are now needed to address the etiology so that better information can be provided for counseling prospective parents.

15. Misconceived conceptions

A search through the scientific literature on the subject of medical errors in IVF yields very few publications, although on several occasions reports in the lay press of IVF mix-ups have stirred public opinion. The news that white couples undergoing IVF treatment were having black babies has been front-page news on more than one occasion. The cases caused great concern amongst the millions of couples who had used IVF. If mistakes are only apparent when a couple has a child of a different color, the question arises: how many errors go unnoticed or are covered up in one way or another?

In the Netherlands, in 1993, a white woman gave birth to two boys, a white one and a black one. Subsequent inquiry into the incident established that the white boy was the natural child of both parents, but the black boy had a different genetic father. In this case the biological father of the black baby did not try to claim his child. An internal inquiry commission at the hospital, completed with an external member with embryological expertise, reviewed the IVF procedures in the hospital in an effort to clarify what exactly went wrong. The inquiry commission concluded that it was impossible to exactly pinpoint the cause of the event. The commission further concluded: "although the commission understands that the IVF procedures practiced are according to the normal standards in Dutch IVF laboratories, it endorses improvement of the current IVF practice". The report further stated: "Because a unique living product comes into being in the IVF laboratory, the procedures in such a laboratory should follow the strict guidelines of Good Manufacturing Practice (GMP), as used by the Pharmaceutical Industry". Since the staff supposed that the error was made somewhere during the process of pipetting or by the insemination itself, they set out to carefully identify all 'GMP' sensitive steps in their procedure. This included all elements where a change of tube or vessel seemed necessary for a sample or suspension, all products of different origin came near to each other and all procedures regulating transfer of products to and from patients. Although the process of identification of GMP-sensitive steps and translation into detailed written procedures proved to be an enormous amount of work, the implementation of many of the practical consequences in daily IVF work went smoothly and did not lead to a substantial enhancement of the daily workload.

During subsequent years other cases of misconceived conceptions became known publicly. In the US, in 1998, in what is known as the Donna Fasano case, a white woman gave birth to two boys – one white and one black. The embryo mix-up occurred at a New York IVF clinic in 1998 when two women were there to have their fertilized embryos implanted in their wombs. A doctor admitted he put some of the fertilized embryos of the black woman, called Rogerses, into a catheter that was used to implant the embryos of Donna Fasano, then 37 years old. The other woman was implanted only with her own fertilized eggs; none of those produced a fetus. The white woman was the unwitting surrogate mother for a black baby. After a "bitter custody battle" the black couple whose embryo was mistakenly implanted into the white woman won custody of the black baby and six months later the Fasanos gave the black baby back to the them.

In another case a switch of embryos occurred at a San Francisco clinic in 2000 and was noticed by the doctors minutes after treating

Ms Susan Buchweitz. The embryos she received were intended for a married couple that underwent IVF on the same day. The embryos were created using the husband's sperm and a different egg donor. The doctors hid the mistake and the patient learned about the switched embryos when the son was 10 months old. This was after the Medical Board of California, acting on an anonymous complaint from a former worker at the clinic, contacted the patient and said there had been a mistake with her IVF procedure. After she contacted the clinic the doctors went to her home and revealed to her what had happened. They also notified the other couple that filed their own fraud-and-negligence case against the doctors. According to court papers, the doctors argued that it would be better to let nature take its course rather than disclose the error, possibly causing the patient to end the pregnancy. In court the doctor's attorney said: "The dilemma he (the doctor) had was that if he told somebody, he had to tell everybody, and somebody would be harmed as a result of it". A family court judge granted Ms Buchweitz temporary custody of the boy and the biological father, twice-weekly custody. How care will be divided in the future would be decided at a later stage. The woman reacted: "It's so ironic the court would ask people who don't know each other to co-parent". The Californian woman was recently awarded $1m in damages.

Other cases of misconceptions were reported recently in the UK. At the Leeds General Infirmary an error became apparent in July 2002 when a white woman delivered twins of mixed race. Two couples – one white and one black – underwent IVF treatment. The white woman became pregnant and gave birth to mixed race twins. Genetic tests established she was their biological mother, which meant doctors had used the correct eggs, but that the woman's eggs had not been fertilized with her husband's sperms as planned. An internal hospital inquiry suggested that the mistake probably occurred either when the samples of sperm were placed in a centrifuge or when they were removed from a storage box immediately before being injected. An inquiry, led by a specialist in risk management, was set up. A report was commissioned two years after the mistake occurred and revealed that other mistakes were made in the same department. One involved the loss of embryos following a failure to check liquid nitrogen in a cryogenic freezer. Another saw the disposal of embryos following an administrative failure. The report included recommendations such as:

- Double-checking patient identification at all stages of treatment;
- Unannounced inspections of clinics;
- Improved recruitment and training of inspectors and staff;
- Setting up an alert system to ensure timely investigation of all incidents.

A specialist in risk management said confidentially that events had led to a "culture of secrecy" and had had prejudicial effect on the authority's ability to carry out its duties in an open and effective way.

The High Court was asked to settle the issue of legal paternity of the children. This will determine which couple will have the right to bring up the children and whether the other couple will have any rights to see the twins. The black man whose sperm was used to fertilize the twins has recently been named as their legal father. The ruling would suggest that legal parentage of children born as a result of an IVF blunder would be awarded to the biological parents.

According to some lawyers the decision in the Leeds case appears to swim against the tide of legal and cultural change, which has in recent years been moving towards an acknowledgement that "what really matters" about families is not genetic relationship, but bonds of care between people who may or may not be biologically related. But in this case, which comes to acknowledge the importance of the biological role, it is hardly conceivable that the children would not ask about their genetic background; full openness is really the only acceptable approach.

In 2002 all centers in the UK licensed to offer IVF treatment were told that they had to double-check the identification of people undergoing treatment and the sperm and eggs at the time of insemination. They were also told to double-check the identity of the embryo and patient during embryo transfer and the gametes and embryos at the time of freezing and thawing.

In October 2002, another IVF mix-up was revealed at a London hospital. A doctor in charge of the IVF clinic at St George's Hospital spotted the error hours after the embryos had been transferred. The error, which happened in April 2002, involved three women – the first of whom had reportedly produced a number of embryos, from which only the best quality pair was chosen. The woman was implanted with her own "poorer quality embryos" while her "best quality pair" went to another woman whose embryos were given in error to a third woman. The women who got the "wrong embryos" have been left "devastated" and "traumatized" after undergoing an "emergency procedure" to have the embryos removed. Dr. Nargund, who was responsible for the clinic, raised concerns about management failures and threatened to report this to higher authorities, then was suspended by the Hospital Authority. The unit was shut down, the trust launched an inquiry into what had gone wrong and the facts were reported to the Health Authority and the Department of Health. Dr. Nargund was deeply upset because the suspension appeared to suggest that she was responsible for the mix-up and for the suspension of the unit's service. Her husband said that she was suspended because she was a whistle-blower. After libel proceedings in London's High Court by St George's Hospital, the NHS apologized to Geeta Nargund and agreed to pay her a substantial five figure sum of damages and costs of more than £100,000.

In August 2001, *The Sun* newspaper reported that a British teenager had discovered he had the "wrong" father after a mix-up at the IVF clinic where his mother was treated. In 1988, the boy's mother and her then husband received IVF treatment at a private hospital in north London. She was delighted to become pregnant, but as her son developed, she began to think he did not look like his father. As the boy grew older, he also began to have suspicions. DNA tests were finally ordered and confirmed the error. However, the boy will not be able to find his biological father, as hospital records can no longer be found. A lawyer specializing in family law commented that there should be a policy of presuming that, if paternity is an issue, there should be an indication for a DNA test right from the outset. If the case could have been solved at an early stage the cost, aggravation and stress of the court proceedings could have been avoided.

The ethicist, John Harris, in discussing assisted reproductive technology blunders argued recently that:

> "While maintaining and insisting upon the high standards from assisted reproductive services where, as it is inevitable in all human affairs errors occur, priority should not be given to the correction of those errors, which may, from the point of view of both ethics and justice, be undesirable and unworkable, but rather address directly the question of what is the best for everyone in their respective circumstances".

PART 2

REPRODUCTIVE MEDICINE AT THE CATHOLIC UNIVERSITY OF LEUVEN (K.U.LEUVEN)

CHAPTER V

SEX WITHOUT REPRODUCTION

In 1972, we started with an interdisciplinary group at the K.U.Leuven to discuss, during evening meetings, the medical, psychological, social and ethical aspects of new technologies, which were introduced for fertility control and infertility. The group included an ethicist, an andrologist, a urologist, a psychiatrist-sexologist and gynecologists. The interdisciplinary dialogues resulted in the publication of the book *Menselijke voortplanting en geboortenplanning. Het paar en zijn begeleidend team* (Human reproduction and family planning. The couple and its counceling team) by M. De Wachter, I. Brosens, P. Nijs et al. in 1976.

There was a need for interdisciplinary dialogue when we were faced in the clinic with the failures of the widespread use of coitus interruptus, also known as "withdrawal" or "being careful", and the disastrous effects of criminal abortion. Was it acceptable to prescribe the pill for a mother of six children? How could she protect herself against the failures of coitus interruptus? Not everybody was happy with the attitude of some colleagues who argued: "Well, it's not permitted, but I will prescribe the pill".

From the beginning it was felt that several anomalies in medical practice were not compatible with both a safe medical practice and a humane approach. How could it be justified that a cesarean hysterectomy was performed, but not a tubal sterilization, when the medical condition of the pregnant woman did not allow any further pregnancy? Similar anomalies were seen in other cases where a major medical reason existed for termination of pregnancy. Why refer these patients to a foreign country when the ethical and practical problems could be discussed here in Belgium? Why shouldn't one strive to find a humane and responsible solution? Certainly, it was not easy to change traditional practice at a Catholic university. However, the regular interdisciplinary discussions of medical practice in such problematic cases were of great help to win the trust of patients, personnel, students and colleagues.

16. How the pill was introduced

The steroid components for oral contraception, or the pill, were developed by the industry in the mid-1950s and offered a new and efficient treatment of gynecological problems such as abnormal menstrual bleeding and menstrual pain. They also offered mankind the possibility of controlling ovulation and, therefore, fertility for the first time. The pill controls both ovulation and menstruation. A menstruation-like bleeding occurs when the intake of the pill is discontinued. With a pill regimen of 21 days on and 7 days off the ovulation remains suppressed while a normal menstrual cycle of 28 days is mimicked.

The pill could also be continued without interruption and, after a few months, all vaginal bleeding would stop for as long as the pill was taken. Jacques Ferin, gynecologist at the Catholic University of Leuven, argued in the late 1950s that if there is no desire for pregnancy there is also no need for menstruation. The new steroids allowed suppression of menstruation by suppressing ovulation. In collaboration with the pharmaceutical company, Organon, he developed the progestogen, lynestrenol, which became the first pill to suppress both ovulation and menstruation. By taking 5 mg lynestrenol (Orgametril[R]) daily a woman achieves suppression of ovulation and within two or three months complete suppression of menstruation for as long as she wants. Orgametril became popular for contraceptive use in Catholic countries like Belgium and France. The product was relatively cheap and women have used Orgametril for many years, and even decades, as a highly efficient method of contraception giving them at the same time full relief from the discomfort associated with menstruation. The relief granted by an amenstrual reproductive life is illustrated by the following two cases.

Betty was a 34-year-old American woman who moved some years ago to Brussels to set up a business. She had been taking the pill for eight years. Before that she had had regular but painful menstruations. In 1977 she came to the clinic to discuss the possibility of tubal ring sterilization. At that time it came to her attention that there was a contraceptive pill which eliminated the necessity of a hormonally-induced menstrual period that was thought to make a woman feel more "normal" while on the pill. She was informed that the pill "Orgametril" had side-effects such as an increase in weight, nervousness and dry vagina. She started the pill with 5 mg daily and after six weeks the dose was reduced to half a tablet daily. Initially she was concerned that she had no more vaginal bleeding, but on the other hand she was happy to be free of the monthly inconvenience. Her weight increased slightly, but remained under control. She continued to take half a tablet daily for 18 years until 1995. When she stopped at the age of 52 she was in menopause and had no more menstrual bleedings. Her weight decreased 4 kg and she started her postmenopausal life with a high bone density. Now in menopause, she claims that Orgametril saved her life.

Monique was 33 years old when she came for a gynecological check-up. She had one child born when she was 22 years old. After breast-feeding she started oral contraceptives, but felt unwell at the time of menstruation and that troubled her busy life. In 1973 she started taking Orgametril at 5 mg daily and felt superb without menstruation. The dose was reduced to half a tablet daily, which she continued until 2002. She had no more bleeding after stopping Orgametril and had a smooth transition into menopause.

A female journalist from the Flemish newspaper *De Standaard* wrote, in 2002, in response to a letter on the subject, that the "amenstrual contraceptive pill" has been the best kept secret for women of reproductive age. The explanation is that Orgametril was used for contraception, although it has never been officially registered for that specific indication. The absence of menstruation was described in the information leaflet as one of the potential side-effects. Orgametril, however, has anabolic side-effects such as weight gain, acne, nervousness, and therefore was not really ideal for long-term use. Moreover, the manufacturers preferred to promote an oral contraceptive that mimics a regular four-week menstrual cycle and priority was given to the development of the 21 days on and 7 days off scheme. Interestingly, in recent years an 84-day regimen or so-called "seasonal" pill has been introduced. With Seasonale[R] women have 4 periods each year, instead of the traditional 13. The US Food and Drug Administration recently granted approval for Seasonale[R] as an oral contraceptive.

The main reason why the pill was morally accepted for contraception at the K.U.Leuven hospital was the human misery that was seen in the clinic with the popular, but unreliable practice of coitus interruptus. The practice resulted in many unwanted pregnancies in premenopausal women of all ages and parity. Women had no protection against the frequent failures of coitus interruptus. In the gynecological ward too many desparate mothers with large families at home were admitted in septic shock caused by criminal abortion. Abortion became legalized in the Netherlands and Belgium in 1981 and 1990 respectively. Today, the low abortion rate in both countries is explained by experts as the result of the comprehensive sex education and family planning programs, which were promoted in both countries.

17. Emergency contraception and the intrauterine device

Emergency contraception

In the 1960s, oral postcoital contraception was introduced. Initially, very high doses of an estrogen were given for five days, which caused many side-effects. In 1982, "the morning after pill" was proposed. It was recommended that within the 72 hours following unprotected intercourse one should take two contraceptive pills twice over a period of 12 hours. The method quickly became popular amongst female students at university.

After I had explained the method during a lecture to medical students a female student called my house in a panic in the middle of the night asking whether she should take the "morning after pill" as she had just had unprotected intercourse. When I said "yes, of course" she ran back to the car and I could hear the metal noise of a car driving off at great speed. Did I approve of the use of an abortive agent?

Today, the use of levonorgestrel alone or in combination with ethinylestradiol (Yuzpe regimen) for hormonal emergency contraception has been approved in several countries. However, in conservative Catholic circles it remains an important issue whether the emergency pill acts by preventing fertilization or by impeding the successful development of the zygote through and beyond implantation.

It is too simplistic to state that pills taken after intercourse should by definition be abortive. The question is whether there is a difference in the mechanism of contraceptive action between the pill taken soon after intercourse and the pill taken for 21 days on and 7 days off? In an editorial published in 1997, Tom Eskes, a professor at the Catholic University of Nijmegen, argued strongly that under both conditions the pill is not an abortive agent and acts by preventing ovulation and not implantation. In a recent review, Horacio Croxatto and collaborators at the Catholic University of Santiago also argued that the pre-ovulatory suppression caused by the emergency pill accounts for the prevention of pregnancy. Studies searching for possible alterations that would take place in the endometrium at the time of implantation found no explanation to support an abortive effect. Moreover, recent studies in animals also cast serious doubts that the use of levonorgestrel as emergency contraception prevents pregnancy by interfering with post-fertilization events.

A different situation, however, occurs when the antiprogesterone drug mefipristone is used. The antiprogesterone directly disrupts the process of decidualization or preparation for pregnancy of the endometrium and, therefore, the process of implantation and placentation. In contrast with the emergency pill, the antiprogesterone drug is more effective when the drug is taken later in the cycle, which also suggests an abortive action. The antiprogesterone has been coined the 'interceptive pill' or 'menstrual regulator', as it disrupts the process of endometrial preparation independent of whether or not implantation has occurred.

The discussion reveals that the search for the contraceptive mechanisms acting before or after fertilization and preventing or disrupting the process of implantation remains fraught with hypothetical conclusions. The analysis of the potential mechanisms of direct and indirect action of current contraceptive techniques on the process of fertilization, implantation and early abortion, attains at best a level of probability, but not absolute proof. Within the same ideological discussion it has been suggested that natural family planning methods carry a risk of interfering with normal fertilization in case the method fails and an old egg is fertilized.

Intrauterine contraceptive device

The spiral or intrauterine contraceptive device (IUCD) was, and is, frequently seen as an abortive method. It is supposed to interfere with implantation when fertilization may have occurred. However, there is also experimental evidence in primates that the presence of an IUD accelerates tubal transport and that unfertilized eggs may be expelled. In humans the transport of gametes is also co-ordinated by the intensity and direction of waves of contractions in the Fallopian tube and uterus. In addition, the IUCD modifies the uterine microenvironment and inflammatory cells may interfere with the fertilizing capacity of the spermatozoa before they reach the site of fertilization in the Fallopian tube.

The potential interference with implantation of a fertilized egg was a reason for not using the spiral, unless there was no other acceptable alternative method available. Moreover, there was an increased risk of pelvic infection and, in case of unexpected pregnancy, even sepsis with the original shield type when the device was left in place. Later it was found that the risk of sepsis was due to the multifilamentous thread that acted as a wick for passage of bacteria from the vagina to the pregnant uterus.

The newest types of intrauterine devices, which are covered with copper or release a progestogen, have greatly improved the method. The mechanisms of action of these devices may also have changed. The release of progestogen acts on the cervical mucus and prevents the migration of sperms into the uterine cavity, while the release of copper interferes with the migration and survival or fertilizing capacity of the sperms. In the absence of direct evidence, one cannot state that the current intrauterine devices act before or after fertilization as they potentially have both effects.

18. Sterilization

Cesarean hysterectomy and research opportunities

One of the main issues in reproductive medicine is the prevention of fetal and neonatal mortality. In the 1960s, weekly multidisciplinary audits in the Department of Obstetrics and Gynecology were started to investigate the causes of neonatal mortality which had occurred and how the mortality could have been prevented. Major causes of fetal and neonatal mortality are maternal hypertensive disease during pregnancy and fetal growth retardation. It became important to understand why hypertensive disease during pregnancy caused fetal growth retardation and resulted in a high fetal and neonatal death rate. It is interesting to see how the clinical research projects in this field were very much determined by the prevailing ethics at that time.

The main aim of the project was to investigate why the maternal blood supply to the placenta was reduced in patients with hypertensive disease during pregnancy. Therefore we needed biopsies from the placental bed to examine the maternal arteries, which supply the maternal blood to the placenta. Initially, a technique was used to obtain biopsies from this site at the time of vaginal delivery. After the delivery of the baby the placenta was located by manual examination of the uterus and after the manual removal of the placenta a piece of tissue was obtained from the zone where the placenta was implanted. After normal delivery such procedure required anesthesia of the patient.

Cesarean hysterectomy in Leuven

The method of biopsies of the placental bed produced useful material, but nevertheless was criticized by two great experts in placental anatomy, Professor Hamilton in London and Professor Boyd in Cambridge. They strongly recommended the examination of intact uteri with the placenta in situ for the simple reason that the placental bed is such a battlefield that fetal and maternal tissues are hard to distinguish on biopsy material and that maternal vessels are disrupted after placental separation. Only uteri with the placenta in situ would allow the anatomical identification of the fetal and maternal structures including the blood vessels. Both scientists were working in the UK and had, with the help of coroners pathologists, collected a large number of intact uteri with the fetus and placenta in situ from pregnant women, who had died by accident and required an autopsy.

Clearly, such uteri from pregnant women with an unknown clinical history were useless for our study. However, there was a more appropriate way to obtain uteri from late pregnancies at the Catholic University in Leuven. Tubal sterilization was at that time not allowed in Belgium, but hysterectomy could be performed at the time of a cesarean section when the uterus was considered to be a sick organ. Such was the case in women with repeated cesarean sections or recurrent fetal losses. Needless to say that a hysterectomy at the time of a cesarean section is a significantly more complicated surgical procedure than tubal sterilization.

The practice of cesarean hysterectomy allowed us to collect a unique series of uteri with the placenta in situ for the study of the utero-placental arteries in hypertensive disease of pregnancy. At Christmas time, in 1964, my brother-in-law, a pediatrician, came with his family to visit us in London. He traveled by car ferry and was able to bring two buckets full cesarean hysterectomy specimens preserved in formaldehyde to the Hammersmith Hospital in London. Today it is amazing to think that he got through customs with his strange cargo.

These specimens allowed us to study the course of the maternal spiral arteries from deep in the uterus to their opening in the placenta in normal term pregnancies and third trimester pregnancies complicated by hypertensive diseases. The study led to the fundamental finding that, in women with hypertensive disease, the remodeling of the uteroplacental spiral arteries is defective and, in addition, may develop atherosclerotic lesions resulting in ischemia and infarction of the placenta and inadequate growth of the fetus.

Termination of early pregnancy by hysterectomy in Bristol

After the findings in late pregnancy it was important to know how remodeling of the spiral arteries started during the early stages of pregnancy. For this part of the study we needed uteri with the placenta in situ from normal early pregnancies.

As abortion was not allowed in Belgium, arrangements were made with Geoffrey Dixon, who was head of the Academic Department of Obstetrics and Gynaecology at the University of Bristol. While abortion for medical reasons was allowed in the UK, it is not uncommon for older women to need a hysterectomy. Instead of performing an abortion by curettage, he proposed to terminate the pregnancy by hysterectomy and removed the entire uterus with the fetus and placenta in situ. In this way a large collection of uteri with placenta from the first trimester pregnancy could be obtained.

The specimens allowed our group to describe, in the early 1980s, the trophoblastic invasion in the human placental bed and the adaptive vascular changes from 8 to 18 weeks of pregnancy.

Tubal sterilization

The first case of tubal sterilization at the Catholic University of Leuven was performed in the late 1960s under dramatic circumstances.

The request came from the parents of a schizophrenic girl. The girl, admitted at an institute for mentally handicapped women, escaped several times to travel to a city on the Belgian coast. After one such trip she returned pregnant. The desperate parents arranged that the baby should be given up for adoption and asked – the father being a lawyer – that after delivery the girl should be sterilized. Three psychiatrists, including a university professor, examined the girl and all three agreed that the mental condition was irreversible and recommended tubal sterilization. The case was discussed in great depth, while other options such as progestogen injections with long-term effect were also considered. Finally, it was agreed with the parents that tubal sterilization was the only solution to prevent further risk of pregnancy. However, there were major problems. Firstly, tubal sterilization was illegal in Belgium; secondly, the procedure had never been performed at the Catholic university hospital; and, most importantly, the mental condition of the girl did not allow one to obtain informed consent. When she was seven months pregnant the girl escaped once more, on a Saturday, from the institute, and on this trip her waters broke. The day after, on the Sunday, she hitchhiked to see her gynecologist at the university hospital in Leuven. She was admitted and, although the medical indication was arguable, the gynecologist decided to perform a cesarean section. This would also facilitate the discrete performance of tubal sterilization. The only person informed, apart from the senior resident, was the head midwife-sister, who directed the delivery quarters. It was obvious that she would notice the unusual procedure. Upon explaining the circumstances to her she agreed with the decision. Her help was most important as she could make sure that nobody else in the operating room, not even the anesthesist, would notice the sterilization procedure. After all, the tubal sterilization was illegal and to perform the procedure without consent could have grave consequences. After the sterilization the gynecologist informed two more people. He made a call to Jean Snoeck, a highly respected gynecologist at the Free University of Brussels and asked whether he had ever performed a sterilization on a woman without her consent. Snoeck replied: "Yes, once on a girl from a center for mentally handicapped people". This answer was already a great relief. The gynecologist also felt it was best to inform his wife as well in case the facts became known and police or other judicial people would be calling at their home. As she was medically trained she could well understand the circumstances and, with the unanimous advice of three highly respected psychiatrists, she also approved of the decision.

In 1969, Marcel Renaer, Professor of Obstetrics and Gynecology and Medical Ethics at the K.U.Leuven, defended the use of sterilization at the National Belgian Medical Council. Legal advisers had difficulties in accepting sterilization because it was a mutilating procedure and, therefore, illegal. Renaer defended tubal sterilization on the grounds that when a woman with several children decides not to have any more children there is no substantial difference between taking the pill until menopause and tubal sterilization.

The case set the stage for tubal sterilization to become accepted for permanent contraception at the K.U.Leuven in the 1970s. Initially, it was done after psychological evaluation in women who had completed their family or had a major reason to request sterilization. Laparoscopic sterilization using mechanical techniques, such as the Falope ring or the clip, was introduced in the mid-1970s and the minimally invasive procedure became in Catholic Flanders, which is the Dutch-speaking part of Belgium, a popular method for permanent contraception.

In search of reversible tubal sterilization

Female sterilization, although essentially irreversible, became increasingly used as a method of birth control. As a result a number of previously sterilized women found themselves in the position of requesting reversal. Particularly at risk were women who were sterilized for medical reasons, or women who were sterilized under the age of thirty or because their marriage was in jeopardy. Some of them bitterly regretted their incapacity for future childbearing. This situation led to an increased interest into research to improve methods for Fallopian tube reanastomosis.

The standard technique of tubal sterilization was to destroy, by resection, a segment long enough to be sure that no recanalization would occur. The goal was to achieve permanent occlusion of both Fallopian tubes. With the introduction of laparoscopy and mechanical techniques, such as the ring and clip, tubal sterilization was less destructive since a segment no longer than 1–2 cm at close distance to the uterus was eliminated. As a result, the more complex distal tubal segment remained intact. Using microsurgical techniques there was a high possibility that the patency of the isthmic segment could be restored. In sterilized rabbits the microsurgical techniques allowed restoration of tubal patency in 100% of the cases and pregnancy was achieved in 95% of the cases.

In clinical practice the success of tubal reanastomosis is dependent upon several factors. Foremost of these is the amount of Fallopian tube remaining after the sterilization. If at least 4 cm of healthy tube is present then pregnancy rates of 60–85% are not uncommon. The highest success rate by microsurgery is achieved after sterilization using the ring or clip method or bipolar coagulation of the isthmic segment. Although reversibility can be high, with the variability of tubal damage and the need for surgical repair, tubal sterilization should continue to be considered as a permanent method of contraception.

Rather ironically, the first demand for reversal of sterilization at the K.U.Leuven came from the young woman who had been sterilized for medical reasons without personal consent.

The young woman was the mentally ill girl described above who had been the first case of tubal sterilization performed at the K.U.Leuven. Some years after the sterilization she was treated with lithium carbonate and her mental state improved considerably. She got married and asked her psychiatrist if she could use the pill for a year or so. The psychiatrist knew that she had been sterilized and so she was told that this may not be necessary and she was advised to go and see her gynecologist. There she was told, half the truth and half a lie, that at the time of the cesarean section the tubes were found to be in a knot and that she could not become pregnant unless the knot was removed. Both tubes were repaired by microsurgery and she conceived twice after the reversal and had two children. At a later stage, however, her mental state deteriorated again. It is known that treatment with lithium carbonate may alleviate symptoms, but is not a cure for schizophrenia.

Why women request reversal of sterilization

The following story illustrates how medical indications for tubal sterilization are relative and can be a cause of regret.

A young woman with renal failure, although she had no children, needed a kidney transplantation and it was advised by the physicians that during the renal transplantation a tubal ligation should also be performed to prevent the "risk" of a pregnancy. It was, however, for the transplantation surgeon, his first tubal sterilization. The kidney transplantation was successful, but soon after discharge from the hospital the patient was referred to us because her menstruations had stopped. Pregnancy was diagnosed. The patient decided to take the "risk" of continuing her pregnancy and had a normal, healthy baby. After pregnancy she developed symptoms of kidney rejection and when surgery was performed to remove the rejected kidney it appeared that not the Fallopian tubes, but the uterine round ligaments had been ligated. Afterwards she received a new kidney, but refused to be sterilized. The outcome repeated itself. She had another healthy baby and kidney rejection occurred again after delivery. At the time of a third kidney transplantation, she had two healthy children and requested tubal sterilization.

In 1977, the gynecologist Robert Winston, later to become Professor Lord Robert Winston at Imperial College School of Medicine in London and today well known to audiences throughout the world for his BBC television series on complex scientific subjects, stayed for a period of one year at the Center for Microsurgery in Leuven to further develop his technique for sterilization reversal. He published, at that time, in the *British Medical Journal* the results of his investigation into why women request reversal of sterilization. The results were based on 103 women who had requested reversal of sterilization.

One hundred and three 22- to 46-year-old women requesting sterilization reversal were interviewed. Only 11 had been over age 30 years of age when sterilized. The mean of term pregnancies at the time of request had been 3 and the maximum number of term pregnancies 7. There were 65 patients who had been sterilized immediately after pregnancy. Pregnancy had been terminated in 37 patients. 3 patients had had 2 abortions and 1 had had 5 abortions. The methods of sterilization had varied. Therefore, laparoscopy was often done to assess the feasibility of reversal. About half of those investigated were regarded as not suitable for reversal surgery. Contraceptive advice given before sterilization had been inadequate in about half the cases. Psychiatrists had advised sterilization in 6 cases and also supported their reversal requests. Unsatisfactory marital relations had been the cause for sterilization in 78 patients. Sexual satisfaction had improved after sterilization in 47, but was less so in 49. The most important reason for reversal request was remarriage in 81 cases. Very careful counseling is recommended before sterilizing young patients, patients with unhappy marriages, or immediately after a pregnancy. An unsatisfactory marriage may be an insufficient reason for sterilization.

The work on reversibility of tubal sterilization was the subject of two international conferences held in Leuven. The proceedings were published in *Reversibility of female sterilization* edited by I. Brosens and R. Winston (Academic Press 1978) and *Reversibility of sterilization. Psych(patho)logical aspects* edited by P. Nijs (Acco 1980).

Vasectomy

Male sterilization, or vasectomy, is the procedure by which the tube carrying sperm from the testicles to the penis is blocked. The procedure was introduced in the same period as tubal sterilization at the K.U.Leuven.

At one stage the use of rings for tubal sterilization inspired a colleague to propose the Falope rings for the occlusion of the vas deferens in men. Hopefully, the rings would make reversal of male sterilization easier. The American company producing the Falope ring instruments was happy to make a short model of the laparoscopic applicator for tubal sterilization. Unfortunately, no preliminary investigations were performed in animals before a first series of men were sterilized with the Falope ring. The experiment in human males was a complete failure. In fact, the ring was inappropriate to occlude a vas deferens. The semen controls after Falope ring sterilization consistently failed to show azoospermia. All men operated on had to be recalled to have the standard procedure of vasectomy.

Reversal of male sterilization, or vasovasostomy, is performed by reattaching the two free ends of the vas deferens. Microsurgical techniques achieve the best results. There are a variety of microsurgical techniques for reanastomosis of the two ends of the vas deferens, with no one type of procedure being significantly better than another. The choice of the exact method is up to the individual surgeon, but microsurgical techniques have much better results than those performed without the microscope. The results of a vasectomy reversal are surgical patency, which means sperms in the semen, and pregnancy. The average patency rates achieved with vasovasostomy performed by microsurgery are approximately 90% using modern microsurgical techniques. However, the pregnancy rates are dependent upon many factors independent of the surgery and average approximately 60%. It has been estimated that the maximal pregnancy rate that can be achieved with vasovasostomy is 67%. A major reason of pregnancy failure is that antibodies to sperms develop in 50–80% of men who have had vasectomies and that these antibodies can agglutinate and immobilize the sperms.

CHAPTER VI

REPRODUCTION WITHOUT SEX

The confrontation between sterile couples and fertility experts became a challenging issue in the infertility clinic. The original attitude was to respond to sterility with adoption or foster parenthood. The fertility team moved progressively towards considering options in addition to the ways of traditional parenthood, such as artificial insemination with donor sperms in the case of male sterility since the 1970s and in vitro fertilization in severe cases of tubal infertility since the 1980s.

19. Donor insemination

Andrology, or the science of dysfunction of the male genital system, was introduced at the university hospital by an endocrinologist affiliated as professor with the Department of Medicine. After a training period at different leading andrology centers in the Netherlands, Germany and the US, he returned to Leuven in 1966 to set up a unit for andrology including homologous insemination and subsequently a program for donor insemination and sex selection.

Donor insemination

One of the most contentious issues for the university and hospital authorities has been donor insemination. Initially patients were referred to an andrology center in Amsterdam, but the services became questionable and expensive. The Belgian patients had to park their car out of sight of the clinic. The poor quality of services in Amsterdam was the main reason that, in 1971, a high-quality program of donor insemination was started at the Catholic university hospital. While the service of donor insemination had departmental approval, it was not officially sanctioned by the hospital director and the story of donor insemination at the K.U.Leuven became very dramatic.

It was the andrologist who personally had to make all arrangements of donor recruitment, appointments, insemination and payments. The andrologist fulfilled the role of a trusted mediator between the donor and the couple. To ensure anonymity, the donor had to enter and leave by the back door, while the couple were waiting in the clinic (sic). Although sperm freezing was already established, the unwillingness of the hospital director to be involved in the service meant that for many years no permission was granted to purchase freezing and storage equipment. Only fresh semen could be used. For in vitro fertilization with donor sperm this sometimes had dramatic consequences, for instance when the donor failed to turn up or when he was unable to produce a sample on the critical day that the eggs were collected and needed to be inseminated. Once, a junior doctor had to rush to the home of the donor pleading for a sample. Even worse, the use of fresh sperm made it impossible to screen adequately for sexually transmitted diseases. Only with the advent of HIV and AIDS, was it finally realized by the hospital authority that the use of fresh semen was totally irresponsible. In 1992, the hospital director approved to buy freezing and storage equipment for the program.

With increasing demand, the recruitment of donors at the Catholic institution also became problematic. The andrologist had to recruit discretely and succeeded in obtaining sufficient donors for his practice, but not for the extra demand made by the IVF program. Moreover, the Cardinal expressed his protest to the dean of the faculty of medicine when medical students in their last clinical year were informed about the possibilities of serving as candidates for sperm donation. The dean objected to the recruitment of medical students as sperm donors. Moreover, he strongly disapproved that cases of donor insemination were discussed in the presence of doctors in training.

In January 1995, the shortage of donors became acute. The dean then suggested that, in order not to upset the Church hierarchy, this problem could be solved by discrete recruitment of candidate donors at an affiliated hospital in Brussels. The samples could be stored in Brussels and, when required, transferred for insemination to the Catholic University Hospital in Leuven. However, the gynecologist disagreed and argued that patients might as well travel to Brussels for the treatment.

Guidelines by the Committee for Medical Ethics

In a first interim report on the ethical acceptability of donor insemination the Committee for Medical Ethics stated, in 1975, that within the teaching of the Second Vatican Council, the praxis of donor insemination can be seen as a responsible assistance to human beings in need for two reasons.

Firstly, reproduction in a human couple is not purely the biological creation of children, but needs to be conceived existentially as a joint engagement for the mutual promotion of human beings, for the education of the children, for service to others and so on. The physical sexuality is, according to the Concilium teaching, situated within the expression of the totally embracing union of love in which the child is conceived. Parenthood is, therefore, not dominantly or primarily biological but should be situated within the totality of the conjugal relationship.

Secondly, biological parenthood is important but clearly secondary to the total values of the couple and family relationship. This principle has already been accepted in Catholic teaching in other fields such as family planning and adoption. The same principle is applicable when donor insemination contributes positively to the quality of the couple's relationship: the unavoidable loss of biological parenthood can be compensated for by the more human quality of couple and family relationship.

Criteria for the selection of the donor were established and included:

1. Genetic screening of the donor, including clinical examination;
2. Psychological assessment, with evidence of mental stability;
3. A minimum age of 25 years;
4. The donor should preferably already be a father.

At that time the committee also recommended separation between the praxis of donor insemination and the responsibility for semen collection and storage. This would have involved the organization of sperm banking.

Many years later, in 1989, the Committee responded to several fundamental objections which emerged, such as the introduction of a third party in the relationship, loss of rights of the child by the anonymity of the biological father, acceptance versus refusal of sterility within Christian tradition, replacement of natural conception by an artificial act and the potential lack of interest in further investigation and treatment of male infertility.

The Committee formulated the following recommendations:

1. The clinical indication should be well established;
2. The couple should be fully informed and agree with all implications;
3. The couple is likely to be able to care for the education of the child.

The practical modalities of the procedure included:

1. Absolute anonymity of the donor;
2. The donor should be investigated for his motives and also have a clinical and genetic examination;
3. Donation is without financial benefit;
4. There should be a guarantee that the male partner agrees freely.

Some members of the Committee took, in principle, a more restrictive viewpoint. This was motivated by the opinion that donor insemination is a grave violation of the conjugal relationship.

A third recommendation, in 1998, took into account that other Catholic universities had stopped the sperm donation program, that intracytoplasmic sperm injection had removed many of the indications for sperm donation and that the small number of cases no longer justified the local recruitment of donors, but foreign sperm banks could be used. However, the Committee remained divided in its advice and recommended that the academic authorities formulate a clear position to remove the persisting insecurity amongst the personnel working at the fertility center.

20. Sex selection

While the andrologist introduced donor insemination in the 1970s, a procedure that was not always wholeheartedly supported by all staff members in his department, he was also one of the first in the world to develop a technique to separate the sperms carrying the X- and Y-chromosomes for preconceptual sex selection.

Control of sex selection has been a human dream for a long time. In the Bible we read "when a woman produces her seed first, she will be carrying a male infant, when a man produces his seed first she will be carrying a girl." Clearly, we should read orgasm for seed. Throughout the centuries the sex of the baby was thought to be determined by sexual activity and innumerable recommendations on timing, position and abstinence from sex were proposed to achieve the desired sex of the infant.

Techniques for sperm separation

In the 1960s, so-called natural methods for sex selection were developed which were based on differences in swimming characteristics between X- and Y-chromosome carrying sperms. The Y-chromosome carrying sperms are smaller and faster, but have less energy. In a less acid environment they would be faster than X-chromosome carrying sperms, while in a more acid environment the X-chromosome carrying sperms would be favored. Recommendations for a boy included coïtus at the time of ovulation and for a girl two to three days before ovulation. Further recommendations included irrigation of the vagina with a solution of sodium bicarbonate, orgasm of both partners at the same time or abstinence for the man from the beginning of the cycle. The claim that coitus at the time of peak mucus leads more often to boys was refuted by a controlled study of the sex of the baby in relationship to the date of ovulation. Other natural methods based on diet therapy also claimed a high success rate and became popular.

More scientific methods were described which attempted to separate the X- and Y-chromosome carrying sperms and to use the X- or Y-fraction for artificial insemination in order to obtain a girl or a boy respectively. The andrologists Arif Adimoulja and Omer Steeno published, in 1975, the technique of sex selection using a Sephadex column for sperm separation. The technique resulted in an enriched fraction of Y-chromosome carrying sperms and was an improvement over previous, so-called natural methods, but was also far from foolproof.

The most accurate method of sperm selection is based on DNA flow cytometry combined with a cell-sorter (Microsort[R]). The method is based on the 2.8% difference in DNA-content between the X- and Y-chromosome carrying sperms. Using a fluorochrome pigment that binds to the DNA-helix, the sperms are separated by laser-light. In comparison with the postconceptual techniques of fluorescence-in-situ-hybridisation (FISH) and the polymerase chain reaction (PCR) after in vitro fertilization this is the only method of sperm separation which achieves 90% accuracy. By combining the flow cytometry and PGD for X-linked diseases an accuracy of 100% can be achieved that the implanted embryo is female. In this way the abortion of a male embryo, whether or not affected, can be avoided.

Who asks for sex selection?

In humans there are firstly medical indications. Amongst the more than 3000 congenital abnormalities there are about 370 that are X-bound or sited in the X-chromosome. They are gene mutants of the X-chromosome. In women, the healthy chromosome compensates for the defective one. In boys, 50% are affected, while the girls are only carriers of the defective gene. Examples are hemophilia A and B, muscular dystrophia of Duchenne-Becker, X-bound mental retardation, retinitis pigmentosa, glucose-6-phophate-dehydrogenase-deficiency, familial congenital hydrocephaly, achromatopsy and the fragile X-syndrome.

After reviewing 127 publications Steeno found that there was not a single paper disapproving of sex selection for a medical indication. In support of the technique are the avoidance of parental distress, the physical and psychological suffering of the child and the social and financial burden required for the appropriate care of the child.

In practice, however, only a small proportion of the requests for planned sex selection are for genetic reasons. In a New York clinic only 2.6% of the requests were for medical reasons. The vast majority of requests from people with a planned sex choice are for social, economical, cultural, personal or even religious reasons. The motivations vary between:

• The wish for a sex-balanced family;
• The wish for a first born of a specific sex;
• The wish for a particular order in the sex of children;
• The wish for a child of one's own sex;
• The economic motivation, particularly in rural areas in Asia: men are needed for agriculture, represent security for later in life, do not need a dowry, continue the family name and inheritance or secure the family business.

It was the pressure from the "social requests" which made the andrologist decide not to continue with the practice of sperm selection. A fortune could have been made as seen by the exploitation of a similar method, which at that time was developed by Ronald Ericsson. The procedure was based on serum albumin gradients and was used in the fertility centers of the chain Gender Clinics. Each clinic had to pay an initial fee of US$ 7.500 and a further 17% royalties on the US$ 500 fee for each treated sperm sample. The technique resulted, in contrast with the Steeno technique, in an *enriched fraction of Y-chromosome carrying sperms. Both techniques were far from foolproof, however, and were severely criticized. Ericsson claimed a success rate of 72%.*

The official position of the Catholic Church

According to the classic Catholic moral teaching, natural intercourse is a must for reproduction. Moral theologians with a personalist view, however, no longer agree. The main issue remains when new life actually starts. According to the classical norms, life starts at the time of the fertilization of the egg by the spermatozoon and the formation of the sex identity, whether XX or XY. Some moral theologians argue that new life requires that the new biological entity establish a "social" contact, which is at the moment there is an exchange of signals between the fertilized egg and the maternal environment, whether in the tube or the uterus. According to others, new human life requires the onset of the neural tube development as the beginning of the central nervous system.

During an interesting table conversation with eminent moral theologians the question was raised whether an anencephalic baby with the cerebral hemispheres completely missing or reduced to small masses should be baptized. The Jesuit professor Richard McCormick, Professor of Moral Theology at Georgetown University responded "no". Monsignor Martens, a theologian at the Catholic University of Leuven, however, would baptize the anencephalic newborn. Without a new divine revelation the question remains unanswered!

Abortion of a fetus with an X-linked disease was, in the 1960s, not acceptable for the Church Authority, but was practiced in many Catholic hospitals. Pre-conceptual selection of sex by separation of sperms was also not acceptable for the Catholic Church because the sample was obtained by the unacceptable act of masturbation.

21. The first Belgian IVF baby at the K.U.Leuven

On July 25 1978, Louise Brown, the world's first successful test-tube baby, was born in Great Britain. The success was the achievement of Dr. Robert Edwards, a physiologist at Cambridge University, who had been working on in vitro ("in glass") fertilization since the beginning of the 1960s. I remember that in 1964, when I was research fellow in the Department of Obstetrics and Gynecology at the Hammersmith Hospital in London, Dr. Edwards came to see the infertility surgeon in order to obtain collaboration for his project of collecting human eggs at the time of ovulation. However, it was difficult in a busy university clinic to plan the surgery at the right time for the mature eggs to be obtained from the ovaries. He found, however, in Dr. Patrick Steptoe, a gynecologist at Oldham General Hospital, a highly motivated collaborator. In addition, Dr. Steptoe was one of the first in the UK to use the laparoscope for infertility diagnosis, which offered a more convenient approach for ovum aspiration than the standard open abdomen surgery. They started collaborating in 1966. However, until 1977, all of the pregnancies resulting from their procedures (about 80) ony lasted for a short time.

The story of Louise Brown is described in detail in the 20th Century History website.

Lesley and John Brown were a young couple from Bristol who had been unable to conceive for nine years. Lesley Brown had blocked Fallopian tubes. Having gone from doctor to doctor for help, to no avail, she was referred to Dr. Patrick Steptoe in 1976. On November 10, 1977, Lesley Brown underwent the very experimental in vitro ("in glass") fertilization procedure.

Using a laparoscope Dr. Steptoe took an egg from one of Lesley Brown's ovaries and handed it to Dr. Edwards. Dr. Edwards then mixed Lesley's egg with John's sperms. After the egg was fertilized, Dr. Edwards placed it into a special solution that had been created to nurture the egg as it began to divide.

Previously, Drs Steptoe and Edwards had waited until the fertilized egg had divided into 64 cells (about four or five days later). This time, however, they decided to place the fertilized egg back into Lesley's uterus after just two and a half days.

Close monitoring of Lesley showed that the fertilized egg had successfully embedded into her uterus wall. Then, unlike all the other experimental in vitro fertilization pregnancies, Lesley passed week after week and then month after month with no apparent problems. The world began to talk about the amazing procedure.

Throughout Lesley's pregnancy, she was closely monitored, including the use of ultrasounds and amniocentesis. Nine days before her due date, Lesley developed toxemia (high blood pressure). Dr. Steptoe decided to deliver the baby early via cesarean section.

At 11.47 p.m. on July 25 1978, a 5 lb 12 oz baby girl was born. The baby girl, named Louise Joy Brown, had blue eyes and blond hair and seemed healthy. Still, the medical community and the world were preparing to watch Louise Brown to see if there were any abnormalities that couldn't be seen at birth.

The success had been a success! Though some wondered if the success had been more luck than science, continued success proved that Dr. Steptoe and Dr. Edwards had accomplished the first of many "test-tube" babies.

In vitro fertilization and embryo transfer was started at the K.U. Leuven soon after the birth of Louise Brown. Ethical problems were raised. Considering the position of the Church that human life begins at conception, the ethical question raised was whether doctors were killing potential humans when they discarded spare fertilized eggs or embryos?

The first Belgian IVF baby was born at the K.U.Leuven in May 1983. The team received no negative comments. One card arrived from someone who called himself president of a society for the protection of the rights of men asking whether the time had come that men could become pregnant.

Why IVF was started at the K.U.Leuven

Leuven was, in the 1970s, a leading international training and research center for tubal microsurgery. Although microsurgery was highly successful for reversal of tubal sterilization, intrauterine pregnancy rates were disappointingly low in patients with severe tubal damage following recurrent pelvic inflammatory disease. The birth of Louise Brown was heralded as a triumph in medicine and science. Sterile women with irreparable blockage of the Fallopian tubes could become pregnant through in vitro fertilization. The hopeless attempts to repair such Fallopian tubes by microsurgery could now be abandoned.

At that time the submission and approval of a protocol by a Committee for Medical Ethics was not required to initiate IVF.

The informal approval of the University Authority came during a dinner when rector Piet De Somer inquired whether we had started IVF. Rector De Somer was the first lay-person to become rector of the K.U.Leuven and, while he did not object to the program, he advised us to keep it quiet.

In December 1982 we had the first ongoing pregnancy. The news was leaked to the press at the time the patient came to the hospital for an ultrasound examination. The next day the expected birth of the first IVF baby in Belgium was front-page news. However, the news was badly received by the dean of the Faculty of Medicine, who ordered that under no circumstances, not even with parental agreement, should the birth be publicly announced. Apparently, the University Authority was anxious not to embarrass the Church Hierarchy in Belgium by the official news that in vitro fertilization was practiced at the Catholic university.

When the expected date of birth passed without press release of the birth some newspapers questioned ironically whether the Leuven specialists had the date of conception wrong. Following this the university released a statement confirming that a healthy IVF baby had been born at the university hospital Gasthuisberg. The identity of the first Belgian IVF baby has remained undisclosed.

As a result of the first IVF success in Belgium the fertility clinic was inundated with requests for treatment from infertile patients. Although IVF was not questioned on ethical or religious grounds in the university hospital, resources were not made available to develop and organize the service. The new technology apparently caused uneasiness amongst some members of the University Authority. For unclear reasons key members of the team were criticized and harassed on spurious grounds by the Faculty Authority and forced to either stop their involvement in the IVF program or to move.

Both the Professor of Obstetrics and Gynecology, who was also Professor of Medical Ethics as well as Rector De Somer continued their support for developing in vitro fertilization at the K.U.Leuven. When, in 1985, Pope John Paul II visited the K.U.Leuven, Rector Piet De Somer defended in his speech the need of "freedom" as follows: *A Catholic intellectual is always positioned at the borderline between what is known and as yet not known. They should be allowed the freedom of committing an error: it is an essential condition for scientific investigators – and for the university as institution – to fulfill their mission. Actual discussions and tensions over moral problems in relation to overpopulation, contraception, certain medical interventions, various theories over the interpretations of particular issues of faith, indicate how delicate the mission of a Catholic university can be; without cease it must try to unite values and truth.*

Spare embryos and cryopreservation

Controlled ovarian hyperstimulation has been used in IVF treatment in order to obtain a sufficient number of eggs for fertilization. The transfer of more than one embryo was found to increase the pregnancy rate significantly. While eggs cannot be selected on the basis of quality, all eggs taken from the ovary are given the chance to become fertilized. Initially the Committee for Medical Ethics recommended the replacement of as many embryos as possible in order to reduce the number of frozen and stored embryos. Such policy, however, caused a dramatic increase in the multiple pregnancy rate. The incidence of multiple pregnancy was around 30%. Moreover, embryo reduction was performed in several cases to reduce the multiplicity of the pregnancy and the associated high risks of neonatal morbidity and mortality. It became obviously clear that the number of embryos transferred should be reduced.

The Committee also recommended the use of the natural cycle in order to avoid the ethical problem of spare embryos.

Attempts were made, in 1993, at an affiliated hospital in Brussels, to perform IVF during the natural cycle in order to avoid the risks of hyperstimulation of the ovaries and, particularly, the ethical problem of the creation of spare embryos. Some successes were obtained with egg aspiration and fertilization in the natural cycle. However, with a success rate of 5% there was no chance that the program could survive. Financial support for the program was not available and after a pilot study of 100 patients the project was abandoned.

When cryopreservation of human fertilized eggs became successful in the mid-1980s the excess numbers of embryos could be safeguarded and transferred during a subsequent cycle when needed. Fertilized human eggs can be stored either on the first day in the pronuclear stage, the second day when the first egg divisions have occurred or later during the blastocyst stage. In the mid-1990s, the Committee for Medical Ethics approved the cryopreservation of fertilized eggs in the pronuclear stage. In 1997, the Committee agreed that priority should be given to the policy of avoiding the risk of multiple pregnancy and the reduction of the number of embryos transferred in a cycle. As a result, of course, the number of spare embryos increased and a large number of embryos were frozen and stored.

By 1999, Belgium had a population of 10 million and had 35 centers offering in vitro fertilization. The number of IVF cycles was around 10,000 a year. Approximately 13,000 embryos were frozen every year and some 5,000 were thawed. The number of frozen embryos rose when the replacement of three embryos decreased between 1994 and 2000 from 50% to 29%. During this period the transfer of two embryos increased from 32% to 52%.

Intracytoplasmic sperm injection (ICSI)

Intracytoplasmic sperm injection was described, in 1992, by the fertility team of the Free University of Brussels (VUB). The technique was discovered rather by accident and, obviously, no experimental work preceded its application in the clinic. The discovery revolutionized the treatment of male infertility and sparked new hopes for couples with male sterility to have children from the partner's gametes instead of having to resort to donor insemination.

ICSI became widely applied in the clinic without formal evaluation of the health of the children conceived with the procedure and before data on safety were available. The technique was used in IVF centers even to the extent of replacing effective treatments and correction of male infertility and to involve cases without male infertility in order to improve the fertilization and implantation rate.

The Committee for Medical Ethics of the K.U.Leuven appreciated that ICSI could replace donor insemination in many cases and recommended, in 1998, that, whenever possible, ICSI should be used instead of donor insemination. At that time, however, safety information was limited to preliminary neonatal data of one center.

IVF mix-up: cover-up never pays off

In the 1990s, the infertility center at the K.U.Leuven was confronted with the dramatic repercussions of IVF mix-ups.

I had responsibility for the IVF program from it's beginning. However, in 1992, the K.U.Leuven and U.C.L had jointly taken over an old hospital in the city of Brussels and I was commissioned to reorganize the Department of Obstetrics and Gynecology. My clinical work was transferred for a period of two years to the Brussels hospital. On my return to the University Hospital in Leuven, in 1994, I was asked to become the director of the IVF program again. The job became, to my great surprise, very difficult. Firstly, I had never in my career experienced difficulty in motivating colleagues and setting up clinical research programs, but this time the collaboration within the team was a great disappointment. Secondly, I was very surprised by the indifferent response of the Hospital Authority when I reported, in 1994, that an error had occurred in the laboratory during the preparation of sperms for in vitro fertilization. The error came to light when, after the preparation of sperm samples and before the insemination of the eggs, the bottle with culture medium was found to contain sperm cells. Clearly, the culture medium had been contaminated during preparation of the sperm samples. Fortunately, the contamination was noticed before the eggs were inseminated. The couples involved were not informed about the incident, but told that for some technical reason a new sperm sample was required. The Hospital Authority was informed, but refused to investigate whether the error was accidental or systematic and could have had implications for patients treated previously. No action was taken except that the technician involved was blamed and relocated.

The internal problems in the IVF team and the attitude of the hospital authority became clear when, some months later, a dramatic error came to light. The news circulated that a patient had sued the hospital for what she called barbaric treatment after an IVF error. Apparently she had become pregnant after IVF treatment, but her pregnancy was terminated because she was told that the pregnancy was abnormal. I was informed by the late Dr. Kamiel Vandenberghe, an eminent sonograher, who was deeply upset that sonography had been abused for misleading this pregnant patient. Being responsible for the IVF program I immediately investigated the case within the team.

The first shattering information was that the hospital authority had instructed my colleagues not to inform me about the IVF mix-up which had occurred during my absence. The mix-up had occurred over a weekend when the embryos were transferred into the wombs of two patients. Immediately after the transfer of the embryos in the first patient the biologist noticed that she had given her the embryos of the second patient. The patients were not informed and in order to avoid suspicion the doctor performed a fake transfer in the second patient. The leftover embryos of the first patient were destroyed. The director of the IVF program was not immediately informed. Probably there was a secret hope that the patient with the wrong embryos would fail to become pregnant. The woman, however, conceived. At that time the hospital authority was informed. The hospital and university authority decided not to inform the couples. A senior obstetrician told the pregnant woman after an ultrasound examination that the pregnancy was

abnormal and that she needed an abortion. The abortion was carried out at
the university hospital.

Apparently the cover-up by the hospital and University Authority created a most damaging "culture of secrecy" that continued to affect the staff, the personnel and the functioning of the infertility center for many years. In spite of multiple requests the University Authority felt it inappropriate to open an internal investigation. Fundamental questions regarding medical, moral and ethical issues were raised but remained unanswered. On which grounds can it be defended that an abortion is performed with incorrect information? Was it acceptable that such an error was not internally investigated and that for many years no guidelines were established as to how to manage, and how to prevent, IVF errors? Why did the hospital and University Authority continue the cover-up on the case for years? Was the policy a manifestation of a slippery slope and the consequence of the ambivalent attitude when a Catholic University Authority allows IVF and at all cost wants to avoid embarrassment to the Church hierarchy?

> At a personal meeting in the office of the rector I learned the argument that in such difficult situations the patient can be assumed to have the right not to know. In 2002, some eight years after the IVF blunder, the rector offered me, through the ombudsperson, the explanation that an investigation was deemed unnecessary for three reasons: firstly, the facts happened too long ago; secondly, the facts belonged to a grey zone; and, finally, under such circumstances and after such a long period the responsibility could no longer be established.

As a consequence, the Leuven university fertility center went through a disgraceful decade. In 2004, the fertility center qualified for the ISO 9001:2000 certificate indicating that in recent years great efforts have been made by the director and his personnel to assure the quality of the IVF procedures. However, the University Authority, never answered the moral and ethical questions regarding transparency and management of an IVF mix-up.

22. Ethical guidelines on IVF

The Committee for Medical Ethics made its first recommendation on IVF in 1984. At that time, 190 patients had been treated and 98 embryo transfers had resulted in 14 pregnancies. The risk of congenital anomalies and the ethical and moral issues regarding spare embryos were the major points of concern. A colloquium in Helsinki reported, in June 1984, that worldwide, 590 babies had been born after IVF-ET. No major congenital abnormalities other than after natural conception were reported. The Committee accepted the use of IVF-ET under the following conditions:

1. The couple should have a stable relationship and have the prospect of providing proper education for the child;
2. The Committee has serious objections against methods which lead to the creation of spare embryos: everything must be done to avoid the creation of surplus embryos;
3. Under no circumstances may the surplus embryos be used for experimental purposes and their survival prolonged;
4. The use of cryopreservation was left undecided as the necessary apparatus was not available at that time.

The recommendations were further adapted in 1989. The diagnosis and indication for the use of IVF were emphasized. The surplus embryos remained a major problem, but IVF should not be stopped for this reason despite the instruction *Donum vitae* of 1987. The Committee proposed the investigation of the use of the natural cycle for IVF or the reduction of ovarian hyperstimulation. In case more than three eggs were fertilized the Committee recommended the transfer of three or maximally four embryos and agreed with the cryopreservation of the remaining embryos. The systematic transfer of all embryos would create an unacceptably high risk of multiple pregnancy.

In 2001, the Committee proposed the following three choices to infertile couples:

1. IVF during the natural (non-stimulated) cycle. This approach reduces the number of available eggs per cycle to one, but may not be applicable in all patients;
2. Careful stimulation which may or may not be followed by the fertilization of a reduced number of eggs. The application of this approach needs to be discussed individually with the gynecologist;
3. Freezing the spare embryos at a very early stage of development with the explicit intention that these embryos are transferred in a later cycle.

Cryopreservation is accepted on the condition that the eggs are used for later transfer, that the transfer may only occur by the agreement of the couple and that, in principle, the transfer of frozen embryos should occur before a new IVF cycle is started. The embryos may be saved for a period of four years, unless the couple makes use of the possibility to extend the period two more years. The agreement is terminated if, during this period, the man and/or the woman dies or the couple divorce or end their relationship.

At the end of the agreement the fertility center will destroy the embryos by thawing. Alternatively, the embryos can be donated to an anonymous couple if the donor was less than 35 years at the time of fertilization.

In 2001, the Committee approved that surplus embryos could be used for embryonic stem cell research. The surplus embryos are donated to a spin-off company associated with the K.U.Leuven and specialized in biotechnological development. In case of patents the couple have to forego the right to financial claims.

Egg donation

In 2001, the Committee also accepted egg donation. According to the Committee, egg donation is ethically acceptable as an important act of solidarity. Solidarity is seen as a positive act when the implications of the donation are fully understood and free and fully informed consent is given. The free donation of eggs to a sterile couple, however, implies that egg donation is done without any right of claim later on and, therefore, the donation is definitive and absolute anonymity must be agreed upon and guaranteed.

Medical indications for egg donation include absence of ovaries, either congenital or post-surgical, infertility with inaccessible ovaries for egg pick-up, premature menopause, genetic defect of the ovocytes and patients with absence of, or very poor, response during ovarian hyperstimulation in IVF. The age limit is set at 40 years at the time of request.

The risks of the procedure for the donor should be well explained and are the same as for IVF including risks such as hyperstimulation, bleeding and infection. The risks for the recipient are minimal at the time of embryo transfer. However, she should be informed that after egg donation there is increased risk of miscarriage, multiple pregnancy, fetal growth retardation, preterm delivery and hypertensive disease of pregnancy.

The initial recommended method was the anonymous cross donation. In practice, two couples, each with a medical indication for receiving an egg, are advised to look for a donor, such as a sister or good friend. Both recruited donors need to be synchronized for hormonal stimulation and egg aspiration. To guarantee anonymity it was proposed that one couple be treated at the university hospital, while the other couple receive hormonal stimulation at an affiliated hospital. The transfer of the embryos could be organized at the university hospital as it was estimated that the chance of both couples meeting would be minimal. Obviously, the arrangements are very difficult. In 2004, the infertility center launched a campaign in a regional newspaper to directly recruit donors with the promise of all costs being paid (by the social security system) and a financial reimbursement of 250 €.

Embryo donation

It would be most appropriate for the Committee that frozen embryos that are not used by the couple are used for donation. Embryos can be stored as long as the agreement is renewed and the costs are paid. When the couple decides not to prolong the agreement the destruction of the embryos is the only remaining solution.

Embryo donation by the biological parents is ethically seen as an act of solidarity. Again, the act should be free willed and the humane approach requires that the biological parents transfer all rights to the child to be born to the "adopting" couple. The Committee argues that full anonymity is required and that both couples should agree to this. However, the Committee realizes that embryo donation can raise problems. Firstly, anonymity may be seen as restricting the rights of the child when it later learns of its origin and wants to know its genetic parents. Secondly, the procedure may look similar to adoption, but the difference is that adoption is a generally accepted alternative for the child that has no parents for its education. In embryo donation the infertile couple achieves a pregnancy with a potential child that biologically originates from a different couple. Such a situation can be psychologically difficult.

According to the Committee there appears not to be a health risk for the donor couple and no increased medical risks for the recipient couple except a small risk at the time of embryo transfer. The risk of genetic defects can to some extent be controlled by the genetic examination of the donor couple.

The program of embryo donation was started after some couples did not agree with the destruction of the embryos and asked whether they could donate the embryos. In practice, although there are a small number of couples who wish to donate their surplus embryos, the demand for embryo donation is low. Surveys have shown that couples attach great significance to genetic parenthood, and this may be one reason that so few embryos are donated.

Preimplantation genetic diagnosis (PGD)

The Committee for Medical Ethics discussed the ethics of preimplantation diagnosis in 1998 and issued a preliminary recommendation at that time. The potential applications of PGD are discussed in detail in Chapter X by Jean-Jacques Cassiman.

The Committee expressed the opinion that PGD was acceptable in some well-defined medical indications, such as patients with severe infertility due to a genetic problem and fertile patients with a genetic indication. Every new medical indication should be presented and discussed by the Committee for Medical Ethics and, for every case, the indication should be discussed by a multidisciplinary team. In each situation the high respect for the human embryo should be measured against the prevention of human suffering. In addition to the principle of weighing the values, caution should be taken regarding the uncertainties and the potential risks of techniques like PGD for the offspring.

CHAPTER VII

ABORTION AND FETAL MEDICINE

In this chapter we describe the first demand for termination of pregnancy at the K.U.Leuven, the position of the Faculty of Medicine in the debate when abortion was legalized in Belgium and the ethical issues of fetal medicine.

When diagnostic tools to evaluate the health of the fetus became available in the mid-1960s, intrauterine interventions were developed in order to treat the fetus affected by life-threatening conditions. The first intrauterine interventions were cases of severe rhesus isoimmunization. Major advances in miniature endoscopy allowed fetal surgery to develop in selected clinical conditions. The Center for Surgical Technologies at the K.U.Leuven became a leading international research center in this field.

The Committee for Medical Ethics at the K.U.Leuven formulated guidelines for abortion in 1989–90 and for fetal medicine in 2001.

23. Abortion

The first request for an abortion at the Catholic university hospital occurred in the late 1960s and was to save the life of a pregnant mother.

The request came from a professor of internal medicine who asked his colleague gynecologist whether he would agree to perform an abortion on a critically ill pregnant patient. She was the mother of four children. Her illness had severely worsened during her fifth pregnancy and she was in a life-threatening condition. The gynecologist asked for more time to reflect. When a week later the physician asked again whether or not he would accept to perform an abortion, the gynecologist agreed with great difficulty and the abortion was performed very discretely in the university hospital.

Legalization of abortion in Belgium

Abortion became a major controversial issue in Belgium when the legalization of abortion was discussed in the 1980s. The first proposals of the early 1970s had been rejected and in 1986 the debate on the legalization of abortion started for the second time. This time the bill would lead to the law of April 1990 allowing for abortion during the first three months of pregnancy.

An ethical position was formulated in 1988 by the Interfaculty Center for Biomedical Ethics and Legislation and was subsequently discussed by the Committee for Medical Ethics. The official position of the Faculty of Medicine of the K.U.Leuven rejected the proposal on the basis of the right of the unborn human life. It was argued that this right should be protected from the moment of conception. On the other hand, a call was made to improve alternative measures, such as:

- Education of the responsibility for his or her own person and for other persons with the inclusion of sexual education;
- Effective assistance in family planning;
- Within the frame of respect for others, providing information on, and assistance with, contraception in order to maximally avoid unplanned pregnancies;
- Effective assistance for women who are in a difficult situation as a consequence of an unplanned pregnancy;
- Improvement of the psychological acceptance and the juridical process of adoption.

The Committee for Medical Ethics considered the approval of the law by parliament as leading to far-reaching permissiveness for abortion in the country, believing that abortion is nothing more than the killing of a new human life. The law would imply that doctors were using their talents not only to help sick people and to protect life, but also to take someone's life away. The Committee considered that such an attitude was totally unacceptable for doctors with a sincere Christian or humanistic attitude.

In 1990, the Committee for Medical Ethics commented on the proposal of a law for the termination of pregnancy in cases of very severe fetal disease that, at the time of diagnosis, are incurable. The proposal allowed the termination of pregnancy without any restriction on the duration of pregnancy or the degree of compatibility with life. According to the Committee members this fell short of infanticide. However, the Committee showed understanding of the dilemma in the presence of a fetal anomaly. In case some groups decided to approve the law, the Committee asked the members of parliament not to approve a law that would not limit the termination, as in surrounding countries, to 24 weeks of pregnancy. The Committee stressed the ethical view that unborn life has an intrinsic value that is essentially untouchable by the age factor or presence of medically diagnosed features or anomalies.

Medical indications

After legalization, the demand for abortion in the university hospital generally came from patients with fetal abnormalities. The obstetrical department had great expertise in prenatal ultrasound diagnosis and the Department of Medical Genetics was well known for pediatric genetics. The demand for termination of pregnancy increased rapidly for women with genetic and major somatic abnormalities of the fetus.

Information on the number and type of abnormalities providing medical indications for abortions at the university hospital remains very discrete.

In vitro fertilization, with the transfer of multiple embryos, also created the major problem of multiple pregnancies. The first case of embryo reduction under ultrasound guidance in Belgium was performed in 1987 at Leuven's Catholic university hospital.

The patient had a quadruplet pregnancy and the pregnancy was reduced by intracardial injection of potassiumchloride to a twin pregnancy. By 1995, approximately 50 cases of embryo reduction had been performed at the university hospital. The risk of miscarriage was 15% in the initial 20 cases, but decreased to 5% in the following 30 cases.

24. Intrauterine interventions

The surveillance of the fetus by modern technology has become an important component of maternity care and is even more important as effective intrauterine therapies are being developed. However, intrauterine surgical interventions are a delicate new field in medicine with many controversial aspects and, therefore, the progress needs to be extremely cautious. The first intrauterine interventions started in the mid-1960s with intrauterine fetal transfusion in patients affected by severe rhesus isoimmunization.

Intrauterine fetal transfusion

Fetomaternal hemorrhage occurs at the time of miscarriage, delivery or an abdominal trauma. In women who are rhesus negative the fetomaternal hemorrhage may result in the formation of antibodies against rhesus positive blood cells. These antibodies can affect the red blood cells of the rhesus positive fetus and as a consequence lead to fetal hemolytic anemia. The risk increases in a subsequent pregnancy and in severe cases leads to fetal anemia and intrauterine death. Fetuses affected by hemolytic disease secrete abnormally high levels of bilirubin into the amniotic fluid. The amount of bilirubin can be quantified by spectrophotometrically measuring absorbance at the 450-nm wavelength in a specimen of amniotic fluid. By serial amniocentesis the evolution of the fetal hemolytic anemia can be followed.

Intrauterine treatment of the anemic fetus started at the university hospital in 1967 with in utero transfusions of concentrated rhesus negative blood. In 1968 we published the first results of intrauterine fetal transfusion in severely affected fetuses at the university hospital. At a time when ultrasound imaging was not yet available we developed, in collaboration with the Department of Radiology, a radiographic technique for the outlining of the vernix layer covering the fetal skin and the gastrointestinal tract. Eight hours after intra-amniotic injection of two radiological contrast media we could visualize, under X-rays, the contour of the abdominal wall and the fetal intestines. After puncture of the fetal peritoneal cavity approximately 50–90 ml packed rhesus negative red blood cells were injected. The treatment was based on the observation that red blood cells injected into the fetal peritoneal cavity were, for the most part, absorbed into the fetal circulation. In 1968, we could report on 19 transfusions that had been given to 12 patients and resulted in 9 live births, of which 3 died during the neonatal period while 6 survived. These 12 patients had a severe degree of rhesus-isoimmunization and had together lost 18 babies.

With the advent of ultrasound the technique of intrauterine transfusion under sonographic guidance became more effective and safer.

The main progress, however, has been the prevention of rhesus immunization by giving all women who are rhesus negative an intramuscular injection of anti-D globulin when there is a risk of fetomaternal hemorrhage. Today, anti-D isoimmunization as a result of the fetomaternal hemorrhage is almost entirely avoidable providing that the prophylaxis is performed at the time of the hemorrhage.

The Center for Surgical Technologies

In 1993, the Faculty of Medicine decided to transform the Center for Gynecological Microsurgery into a training and research Center for Surgical Technologies. The center was designed for training programs in the new endoscopic techniques for different surgical disciplines. The aim was to provide opportunities for practical training in the expanding technology of endoscopic surgery. Many gynecologists and surgeons in practice, who had not received training in endoscopic surgery during their residency, received additional training in endoscopic surgical techniques.

The facilities of the new Center for Surgical Technologies created, in addition, the opportunity for collaborative research with surgeons of different disciplines. At the same time, the obstetrician, Kamiel Vandeberghe, had established, in collaboration with the Department of Genetics, a highly experienced unit for prenatal diagnosis. The collaboration between the Department of Gynecology and the Department of Surgery was a unique opportunity to become involved in experimental intrauterine fetal surgery. Very few centers in the world at that time were involved in fetal surgery, and most of the work had been done by open surgery. The use of the endoscopic approach within a multidisciplinary center of experimental surgery allowed for the exploration of, and the development of, new techniques for correcting abnormalities diagnosed by ultrasound in the fetus.

In 1993, a multidisciplinary team including a visiting pediatric surgeon, a gynecological resident, and the dedicated personnel of the laboratory for microsurgery initiated experimental endoscopic fetal surgery.

It was of major concern that any interventional technique should be extensively investigated by experimental work before being applied to patients. Even more importantly, the clinical indications and selection of patients should be very carefully and scientifically established. Informed consent and full transparency were key issues.

The clinical application of intrauterine fetal surgery could indeed backfire when, as a result of surgery, the fetus survives but remains handicapped. The open, scientific approach also prevents any suspicion or criticism that the survival of a handicapped fetus motivates the team to propose surgery rather than termination of pregnancy at a Catholic university.

The modern imaging techniques and video-endoscopic microsurgery offer new hope for the future of fetal surgery. The research at the center and the clinical applications are described in detail in Chapter X by Jan Deprest.

25. Ethical guidelines for fetal medicine

Pregnancy care includes the care of the fetus as a growing new patient. As the prenatal diagnosis by genetic testing and imaging techniques improves, fetal therapy is increasingly confronted with ethical dilemmas when conflicts arise between the well-being of the mother and the well-being of the fetus or, as in the case of multiple pregnancy, between the well-being of a healthy and a diseased fetus.

The ethical dilemma

The Committee for Medical Ethics recognized the ethical dilemma at an early stage and presented, in 2001, the following considerations and recommendations after ample consultation with experts within the hospital and the university.

- Prenatal diagnosis can lead to very valuable reassuring findings for the patient. Moreover, it is intended to lead to a diagnosis of disorders for which an effective treatment is available. It can also lead to a situation where the interruption of the pregnancy is requested by the patient. The interruption of the pregnancy is evidently against the ethical recognition of the value of unborn life and against the solidarity between the strong and the weak. Moreover, fear exists that it may be the onset of the slippery slope with unforeseeable and far-reaching consequences. One fear is that the abortion of a severely handicapped fetus may lead to the active euthanasia of severely handicapped newborns. The risk of a slippery slope also exists in the absence of objective criteria to make the distinction between light, moderate, severe and extreme types of handicaps or malformations. Ultimately this may lead to a change of opinion in society against the handicapped, where at present the parents of handicapped children can count on a degree of compassion and support from society. Will they in the future be blamed for not having used modern technologies and not having prevented the birth of a handicapped child? As a consequence the world of expectations is changing: some feel it as a moral obligation that the child, at least physically, is as healthy as possible and that medically everything should be done to this end. Whatever is decided by the parents it is important to realize that every decision, even the decision to interrupt the pregnancy, is taken with the deepest wish for a child. The confrontation with the bad news is obviously a most tragic moment for the parents and their decision is to be respected, although it may be questioned.

• The Christian health care community is faced with the dilemma varying between a radical rejection of the request, as proposed by the Church Magisterium (Evangelium vitae nr 63) and a radical negation of the problem. It can lead to the secret practice of a purely technical solution and refusal to recognize that a problem exists.

• The Committee realizes that if it is difficult to openly or publicly discuss the problem as this could lead to an unhealthy practice amongst doctors and midwives.

A Christian-ethical clarification

The Committee states that it is hard to accept secrecy as an authentic Christian attitude. They realize that suffering and defective conditions in modern society are not readily accepted and are, for some, unacceptable. The Christian tradition has always included the fight against suffering. Assisting people in their search for the essence of their suffering can be a way to fight against suffering. Christians believe that in the life of Jesus Christ they find an answer to the search for the essence of human suffering and shortcomings.

Abortion is ethically evil but, in the tragic confrontation of the human being with suffering and shortcomings, can be an acceptable evil and an ethically justifiable choice. Therefore, it follows that in all openness and transparency, the choice of the patient should be respected. The great secrecy surrounding these tragic confrontations is inappropriate and needs to be replaced by a humane and creative culture of assistance. Therefore, the Committee for Medical Ethics has formulated a series of principles and words of advice.

A collaborating relationship

The fundamental principle is that the relationship between doctor and patient is based on trust and open dialogue. At the moment a sort of swing movement takes place from one extreme, the excessive paternalism, to the exaggerated emphasis of the autonomy of the patient or, in this instance, the autonomy of the parents. The option of collaboration, which has been the basis of the advice of the Committee for Medical Ethics, represents a road between both extremes. In fact, the road between involves not only the parents but also the unborn child. All three are necessary for the optimal care of pregnancy.

Ethical principles

Human beings are part of an imperfect world in evolution, with self-renovating mechanisms, even in our genetic material. Some innovations are beneficial, others are unfavorable. Congenital defects are to some extent the price we have to pay for the diversity of the human community. Therefore, it is the duty of the community to take charge of the handicap or disorder of an affected child and to reduce the burden for the parents as much as possible by adequate support.

The fact is that we are faced with an ethical dilemma, by which some values will inevitably be offended. Even when we refuse to make a choice the refusal is a decision pro or contra one of the elements of the dilemma. Whatever can be used under certain circumstances in favor of an abortion there always remains the argument against what is the ethical significance of the unborn life. However, it should be recognized that the unborn life is not the sole value. Other values are also ethically relevant.

The primordial character of the moral obligation allows exceptions in extreme situations. This does not mean that the duty against the unborn life is not compulsory or that respect for the human embryo or fetus depends on the facultative expression of our general respect for human life.

Whatever the motivation of the choice for selective abortion, we are not exonerated from the moral evil of destroying unborn life. It remains an ethical choice in a quasi-impossible conflict, whatever choice the parents may make after the bad prenatal prognosis. In cases where the parents choose selective abortion the decision may well be motivated by their concern for humanity or to preserve other important values.

Guidelines

The proposed approach allows for a careful balance of values and requires a very dedicated service for the couple. It implies a profound solidarity with handicapped children and children with chronic disorders. The solidarity of the community is to support the parents. In the event that an untreatable disorder is diagnosed the responsible doctor's duty is to evaluate, together with the parents, the severity of the disorder and to decide whether or not an abortion is medically indicated. However, it should be remembered that a handicapped life represents its own value in a caring society. Of utmost importance is the humane approach in prenatal diagnostics. As long as no efficient therapy can be offered, the caring approach remains the most valuable alternative.

The caring approach should be present at all stages of the prenatal diagnosis. Information on the procedure, the risks of the procedure, the false positive and false negative results and the feasibility of treatment and its uncertainties need to be provided to the patients. Therefore, collaboration between different disciplines is of crucial importance. This approach demands a highly dedicated team to offer the patients the best possible information, organization and support throughout a most difficult period. It is clear that such an approach is only feasible when there is full transparency and trust between the couple and the professional, caring medical team.

CHAPTER VIII

PERSONALIST MEDICAL ETHICS

Maurice De Wachter is a consultant in bioethics. Before retiring he directed the Institute for Bioethics in Maastricht (1984–1995). Previously, as principal investigator at the Center for Bioethics, he was research professor at the Université de Montréal, taught medical ethics at McGill University (1979–1984), as well as at the Faculty of Medicine and Dentistry, Nijmegen (1974–1978). Between 1968 and 1974 he lectured on theological ethics at the Catholic University of Leuven, and was a member of the "Fertility and Sterility Unit" at the Obstetrics-Gynecology Department. He is a founder of the European Association of Centres of Medical Ethics (1985) and two-term past President of the Association (1992–1998).

Marcel Renaer, who retired in 1983 from his appointment as Professor and Head of the Department of Obstetrics and Gynecology at the Catholic University of Leuven, has dedicated his entire professional life to bring his department in line with leading university departments in the Anglo-Saxon world. The starting point in his endeavors was always with the young and he quickly gained enormous respects as an enthusiastic undergraduate and postgraduate teacher. His deep concern for his patients and the application of the highest standards of care are reflected in the responsibility he undertook in the teaching of Medical Ethics. Marcel Renaer fully appreciated that an academic department in clinical medicine is judged not only on the quality of its teaching but also on the reputation of its research. In addition to his own considerable efforts, over the years he recruited like-minded postgraduates to form a team of basic and clinical scientists whose research results have gained international acclaim and admiration. Amongst many other awards, the conferment in 1975 of Honorary Fellowship of the Royal College of Obstetrics and Gynaecology in the UK is a conspicuous recognition of his achievements.

26. A theory of personalist medical ethics at the Catholic University of Leuven

Maurice De Wachter

*'Il n'est qu'un seul point de départ sûr et solide,
c'est la valeur objective de la personne
envisagée dans sa réalité complète et totale.'*
(L. Janssens, 1939)*

This section and the following one are concerned with 'Personalist ethics and reproductive medicine'. Like the other sections of this book, they address questions of sex and reproductive medicine, but then from a strictly ethical viewpoint. Consequently, criteria for the selection of materials are clear. Personalist ethics will be presented only in order to enable the reader to perceive applications in the field of medicine. On the other hand, personalist ethics applied to other fields with say social, political, economic or environmental issues, will not be developed. Although it is certainly accurate to say that the experience with social ethics based on personalism inspired Louis Janssens to apply the same approach to marital and sexual ethics[1]. Furthermore, personalist ethics applied to fields of medicine other than sexuality and reproduction (e.g. writings about pain killing, organ transplantation, euthanasia), will only be covered insofar as they would support or clarify reproductive ethics. Consequently, there are two sections. First, the current section which is about personalist ethics at the K.U.Leuven, more particularly from the viewpoint of a theory, its origin, its development and its place in today's personalist theories. Then, the next section is about personalist ethics applied to reproductive medicine. For both areas I shall offer representative material on this significant project in medicine and ethics during the second half of the twentieth century.

The founding father: Magister Louis Janssens

European personalism flourished in the 1930s, especially in France and Germany, attracting the interest of a young doctor in theology at the Catholic University of Leuven. His research brought him in touch with a significant group of thinkers in Western traditions for

---

 * *"There is but one certain and solid point of departure, that is the objective value of the person envisaged in the totality of his or her own reality".*

whom the value of the person is basic. He chose to write his dissertation for the degree of "magister" on Emmanuel Mounier's social personalism. There, he clearly outlined his concept of the human person. The very title "Personne et société" (1939) is revealing: person means people together, in groups and institutions. Louis Janssens (1908–2001) thus became the founder of personalism in Leuven. Already, by 1939, he had made it known that, for him, the value of the person considered in his/her complete and total reality, was the only safe and solid starting point for ethics. At first, he applied this approach to social ethics, later to the theology of marriage and sexuality, then to health care and medicine, in particular to procreative issues. By making the concept of the human person central, he replaced the static and a-historical concept of biological nature and natural law by a dynamic and historic concept of the person[2]. One of his major contributions was the rather innovative plea for artificial insemination in 1979. In that article he described personalism in terms of eight fundamental components of the human person integrally and adequately considered. Those components became, then and there, the mantra of Leuven personalist medical ethics. They are, rightly, perceived as adequate foundation of an anthropology in general.

It was probably during the early 1950s, at the time when the ovulation inhibiting contraceptive pills appeared, that Janssens gave his full attention to medical ethics, more particularly to issues of sexuality, marital relations and procreation. He was not the first one to do so. Already, by the 1930s German personalists such as Dietrich von Hildebrand (1929) and Heribert Doms (1935) had explored an experiential and personalist approach to marriage and sexuality. Their focus was on two major themes: the definition of marriage as an intimate communion of spouses in marital love, and the relational meaning of intercourse. In the 1950s, Janssens gave his full attention to these very themes in publications on marriage, the family, birth control, and later fertility and sterility[3]. One theme prepared him, so to speak, for the next one. His innovative insights into marriage as a "covenantal" life and his conviction about the "embodied" person made him encourage the cultivation of human sexuality within the couple. Courageously yet cautiously he first presented hormonal contraception as licit in exceptional situations. The pill, he argued, was only doing what a woman's organism naturally did during lactation, namely suppress ovulation. Chemical intervention can be justified "when one intervenes to assist natural mechanisms which are defective or to correct pathological situations"[4]. Ten years later he was of the opinion that contraception was a matter to be left entirely to the judgment of the conscience of spouses. Indeed, "man himself (autonomy) must endeavor to elaborate concrete moral norms according to available data of experience, that is, according to the acquired degree of knowledge of the laws and values of human sexual relationships"[5]. In a remarkable contribution in this volume, a gynecologist, Janssens' colleague and friend, Marcel Renaer, bears witness to their collaboration in those early days. The judgment of conscience, in the case of contraception, was to be enlightened by indications of efficacy, impact on intimacy, abortifacient effects, and involvement of both spouses in their struggle for "responsible parenthood"[6].

Around 1960, with the fresh wind of *aggiornamento* blowing through the Catholic Church, the Second Vatican Council (1961–1965) offered a unique opportunity to present personalist views for inclusion into authoritative Church documents. Such views were taken to Rome by colleagues of Janssens and by several Belgian bishops. In 1965, the Council fathers approved by an overwhelming majority "that spouses must determine the moral character of their activity according to *objective criteria based upon the dignity of the human person*". Additional suggestions for making a reference to the nature of the acts of the person, brought about the final formulation as '*objective criteria based on the nature of the human person and his acts*' (Gaudium et spes, 1965, nr.51). The official commentary on this expression reconfirms the personalist view when it states that "by these terms it is asserted that also the acts must be judged not according to their merely biological aspect, but insofar as they pertain to the human person integrally and adequately considered"[7, 8]. Janssens' colleagues, Victor Heylen and Philippe Delhaye, as well as the Belgian bishops and cardinal Leo Suenens won a major victory for the texts which Janssens had prepared for them on their mission to the Council. Nevertheless, Janssens found out later that, once the Council was over, the Roman theology remained the basis for official Church documents on sexuality and family. All in all though, he was quite pleased with the result.

During the next ten years, Janssens would apply the conceptual frame of these eight components of the human person to sexuality and reproductive medicine. The result was his '*magnum opus*', the

article of 1979 on artificial insemination. It seems reasonable to
assume that Janssens, in return for the official approval of personalist ethics by the Council, gave full recognition to *Gaudium et spes*. The
twenty page article on Artificial Insemination contains no less than 60
references to that conciliar document. "In this article", Janssens said
later, "I more amply developed the dimensions of the human person
and indicated how they are mentioned in the conciliar documents,
especially in *Gaudium et spes*"[7]. Obviously, Janssens wanted to mark
the conciliar change in favor of personalism in marriage, over and
against the merely biological norms presented in another rival document based on the so-called "Roman theology". That proposal stated,
for instance, that masturbation performed for artificial insemination
was intrinsically evil, and artificial insemination was rejected as
totally immoral[3].

Twenty years later, when Janssens was well into his eighties, he
repeated the eight components, but now in a different order and in
a different interpretation: component six becomes component eight.
In 1979, component six read as follows: 'created after God's image
human persons are called to know and to love God'. In 1999, component eight read: 'human persons are fundamentally directed
toward God.' Not much attention seems to have been given to this
change, but Janssens must have had a reason for it. The context of
the two articles was, of course, different. In 1979, it was about artificial insemination, and point six was developed in terms of spouses
walking the paths of married life, trying to answer God's call. In
1999, he put this call in the broader context of all of moral theology
whose task it is 'to explain how, according to our Christian revelation, our relation to God affects all our doings'[7]. But was the difference in wording simply due to a difference of context? One wonders who or what exactly he was after. True, others too have
changed the order or tied several components together. For instance,
J. Selling changed the order of presentation so that subjectivity,
which was always the first component in Janssens' listing, now
appeared only in the sixth position. "I have done this", Selling
explains, "in order to counteract the Western philosophical preju-
dice toward the subject"[9, 10]. Or, P. Schotsmans reshaping the eight
dimensions into three basic value orientations, as we shall see
below.

Anyway, here are, in brief, the eight essential components of the
human person, in the order of Janssens' last publication[7]:

1. A person is a subject, a moral agent called to self-determination;
2. A person is a subject in a body;
3. Because of the materiality of the body, a person is a being-in-the-world;
4. Persons are directed to each other: the child only becomes a moral subject through others;
5. We are social beings because of our openness to one another, but also because we need to live in social groups with appropriate structures and institutions;
6. Human persons are characterized by historicity, by the history of a personal life and a socio-cultural milieu;
7. Persons are equal, yet each is an original, unique subject;
8. Human persons are fundamentally directed towards God.

Finally, with his feeling for how ethics ought to work, he sums it all up as follows: "For a judgment on the moral rightness or wrongness of an action ... we must consider the whole action with all its components and examine whether or not this concrete totality is promotive of the human person adequately considered in himself ... and in his relations ..."[7].

At this point, we might try to define the meaning of the words "adequately" and "integrally" in the expression "the human person adequately and integrally considered". We may, thereby, also understand the link between the two words and the eight components listed above. The term adequacy seems to indicate that "a moral evaluation or judgment should seek information with respect to all the components ... constitutive of the human person"[11]. All of them need to be considered 'even and especially when it is not immediately evident that one or another of those dimensions may be relevant to the consideration'[12]. The term integrally indicates the concern personalists have for the 'interrelatedness of the various components'[11]. In sum, then, all components together are needed for a comprehensive judgment on the human person's responsibility.

'Janssens' elaboration of a foundation for personalism has proved widely influential in contemporary theology'[13]. Not only is it perceived as the best elaboration of the Second Vatican Council's criterion concerning decisions of sexual morality, but also as an adequate foundation for an anthropology in general[14, 15].

The need for a theory of personalist ethics

The concept of the person was, and still is, open to a great many definitions and interpretations. Therefore, anyone choosing the person as the absolute and ultimate norm in ethics, starts with a serious problem: confusion due to too much variety. Even within Catholic moral theology personalism admits of at least three versions. Common to all three is the acknowledgment of the person as the basic and central notion in ethics, as well as the recognition of the person as a union of bodily and spiritual components. In the first version, moral reasoning remains deductive in order to confirm and further legitimize previous norms. The second version 'reasons' in terms of proportionality and weighs personal values gained against values lost. Depending on this calculation, previous positions may be changed. The third version builds upon awareness through intention and creative conscience. This version wants to embrace human reality in its fullest. Grabowski[13] speaks of rival personalisms in twentieth century Catholic sexual ethics, due to divergent understandings of the key concepts of "person", "nature" and "sexuality and their interrelationships". The three protagonists are Louis Janssens, Paul Quay, and Karol Wojtyla, each of them with rather divergent understandings, indeed.

Janssens tenaciously pursued his insights in the value of the person. He built a framework throughout the many decades he was involved in ethical decision-making in social ethics and in medicine. The list of eight components meticulously put at work in the article on artificial insemination of 1979[3, 7], was rendered in a mere 30 lines in his last article of 1999. But, to call either one of these two instances a theory would, probably, be an overstatement. In both cases the eight essential components seem to be instrumental, a protocol for the elaboration of his argument. In the first case, in 1979, they converge in order to justify artificial insemination; in the second case, in 1999, they show their integration into *Gaudium et spes*, the personalist Church document on marriage. Still, many hidden implications of the eight-component framework remain to be unfolded. This, so it would seem, is a task for those who follow Janssens. Otherwise, there is a danger that such a framework is used as a master key to solve all medical problems. Instead what is needed is another mastermind. Surely, to follow in Janssens' footsteps by doing for other issues what he did for artificial insemination, can and must be done. But, over and beyond that, one is still looking for a more universal, albeit more abstract, theory. Several colleagues and disciples of Janssens have made efforts to identify and meet this need. Wisely, they also look outside for help from distinguished philosophers who have addressed personalism more theoretically. They know that the frame of eight components is not supposed to function as a magic master key. Janssens would never have wanted it that way.

It seems then that, since the founder left, two things have been done: repeating the same exercise over and over again, and simultaneously building a theory. This is a huge task. Janssens himself did the former with great mastery. He did not, however, build a theory. Why? One may presume that he did not feel the need to build a theory because he had one: the traditional and classical moral theology. True, he used that tradition critically; for instance, by not submitting to the so-called 'Roman theology' and to nineteenth-century neo-scholastic interpretations of Thomas Aquinas[3]. Instead, Janssens went back to the angelic doctor himself. There he found enough inspiration to develop a phenomenological concept of the person. Thus, he created a framework with an underlying theory. Since it is unlikely that many would be able to repeat such a return to the sources, we understandably try to build a theory in a contemporary phenomenological style. And, try we must. However, it will take a true mastermind to build a fully fledged theory of personalist ethics.

Again then, what has been done thus far? In the field of personalist medical ethics, several of Janssens' students and colleagues have taken initiatives in two areas. The first is in the area of building a theory of personalist ethics (see below passages on J. Selling, B. Johnstone, and P. Schotsmans). The other is in the area where applied ethics and theory building interact.

Joseph Selling makes several points towards theory building. Firstly, he mentions the need for more philosophical rigor regarding 'the absolutely essential demand for interpretation of experience'[17]. What Thomas calls the *'cognitio per conaturalitatem'* meant for Janssens, the knowledge coming from personal experience. Directly such knowledge would originate from personal experience, indirectly from the experience of others, and in our days from the knowledge gathered by disciplines and sciences that study human experience. Hence, Janssens' keen interest in the human sciences, and his respect for 'serious research'.

Secondly, Selling explicates that the notion of person functions as the ultimate criterion for defining all subsequent ethical concepts, for instance good and evil; and that the notion of person implicitly suggests an appropriate method[9]. For the notion of person to function as criterion, it "must be determined as comprehensive and as comprehensible as possible. Personalism as a philosophical system, is fundamentally phenomenological in character and is based upon descriptions of our observation of, and participation in, reality, as opposed to being based upon 'reality-in-itself'"[9]. Such personalism is continuously open to new experience and insight by the person, rather than to remain static and closed. It can be grasped only 'within the horizon of historical consciousness'[9].

Thirdly, Selling points to proportionate reasoning as an instrument for dealing with good and evil in decision-making, which needs to be clarified and justified[17]. He approaches this theme 'on the proportionate reasoning and the concept of ontic evil' in 2002[18]. Selling here describes in detail how Janssens' understanding of the principle of double effect, combined with a sense of priorities leading to the choice of a lesser evil, deepened into what the Magister himself called a sense of proportion[18]. Selling further outlines the concept of 'ontic evil' which pervades all of our choices, and which Janssens ascribed to our temporality, spatiality, sociality and sin[19].

> "The only really balanced way to perform a moral analysis is with a sense of proportion; or of due proportion, a term coined after Thomas' *debita proportio*. Proportionality is not about acts; it is not about consequences or effects. It is about the ability and the willingness of the human person to embrace an end worthy of being called human and to commit oneself to achieving it"[18].

This repristination of the authentic insight of Thomas about the morality of human activity is not easy to follow. According to Selling 'the real challenge of his (Janssens) thought is appreciated by the relatively few who try to understand him'.

Brian Johnstone critically describes 'both the successes and the limitations of the personalist project in moral theology'[16]. He is of the opinion that this project 'which sought to correct and transform moral theology within the tradition, was fundamentally correct in its basic orientation. There remain, however, serious questions which have yet to be answered'.

For Johnstone, Janssens was 'a notable pioneer' and 'it could scarcely be expected that all problems would be solved from the beginning. If the validity of the new paradigm is to be secured, any unanswered questions need to be dealt with.'[20]

Johnstone himself surveyed the shift from physicalism, where the moral norm is derived from certain structures of nature, faculties or acts, to personalism. He supports the project but has questions about several points in personalism. He asks, for instance: 'What exactly is the status of these dimensions? ... There is no clear explanation ... in Janssens' later writings nor in the writings of those who follow him on this point'[20]. In other words, how do the components interrelate and what is their normative value?

Another question concerns the list of eight dimensions: is this list a description, an ontology (i.e. a theory on being) or a hierarchy of values? Or again, why is there no univocal definition of the notion "the person integrally and adequately considered"? As for the relevance of biological and/or personalist aspects, Johnstone believes that 'solutions to particular problems are based on what appear to be rather *ad hoc* appeals to dimensions of the person; for instance ... the well-being of persons and their relationships can outweigh biological objections against artificial insemination by donor (AID)'[20].

Finally, regarding proportionalism, Johnstone wonders if there is 'any particular personalist character about proportionalism as such"[20]. He understands, though, why personalism and proportionalism often find each other: "the consideration (of) the totality of the dimensions of the person, and of the human reality" calls for "some way of dealing with the multiplicity of factors and the possible conflicts. The encompassing notion of proportion provides this"[20].

Paul Schotsmans repeatedly addressed the need for theory building in personalist biomedical ethics. He insists on two points. One, 'the personalist approach offers a relational foundation for medicine as a healing profession ... and (two) it presents an ethical framework for the integration of new developments in medicine'[21].

Regarding the first point, Schotsmans brings Janssens' eight components together into three fundamental value orientations. These value orientations are: uniqueness, relational commitment and solidarity. They ought to guide the healing profession in its rapport with patients. Together the three orientations endorse the personalist criterion needed to judge human acts. Acts are good if they are truly beneficial to the human person adequately considered. Elsewhere,

Schotsmans puts this criterion into a larger context and calls it 'an instrument for the responsible functioning of our conscience, ultimately the basis of the justification of our action'[22]. In the Christian tradition it is clearly understood that 'every unique human being has to respond for his life by taking up full responsibility before himself, the other, the society, and God'[22].

The second aspect, namely personalism as a frame of reference that helps to integrate new developments such as in vitro fertilization and preimplantation genetic diagnosis will be developed in the next section on reproductive medicine proper.

Complementary investigations à la Ricoëur

It is worth noting that no major philosopher at the Catholic University of Leuven was part of the development of personalism. Several colleagues of the Philosophical Institute supported Janssens' endeavor, but no contribution on a purely rational basis seems to have been made. But, then again, 'medical morals' as it used to be called in the Catholic world, was mainly exercised by theologians. This meant a discipline where reason was looking for clarification by faith and, conversely, where faith was searching for intellect. To work with reason and intellect only was, for the theologian, equal to stepping outside the boundaries of theology. For the philosopher, it would mean to invade a field of theology, overstepping his strict competence. Would this explain the absence of philosophers? Furthermore, the issues at stake were about the moral theology of marriage, sexuality and procreation. Still, one wonders what would have happened, in terms of building a theory, if closer collaboration with philosophers had taken place, as it did with academic colleagues of Janssens in the faculties of medicine, such as J. Ferin and M. Renaer, and even in faculties like psychology and law. Whatever philosophy was integrated in Janssens' personalism seems to have come from his own studies of several philosophers. He was familiar with Henri Bergson, with the French personalists Emmanuel Mounier, Gabriel Marcel and Jacques Maritain, with Emmanuel Levinas and Paul Ricoeur, as well as the German personalist Max Scheler. He knew the existentialists (Martin Heidegger and Jean-Paul Sartre) and phenomenologists (Maurice Merleau-Ponty). However, not one of those philosophers played a leading role in the construction of personalism at Leuven.

Paul Ricoeur, on the other hand, happens to have repeatedly addressed personalism, its strength and its weakness, its permanent appeal, its cycle of presence-disappearance-reappearance, a recurrent pattern which, paraphrasing Mounier, he calls necessary if personalism is to perpetuate itself as a movement. It would seem then that the guest editor of *Ethical Perspectives* rightly included Ricoeur's 1990 article in the thematic issue on personalism in Europe[23]. In the article 'Approaching the human person' Ricoeur makes use of contemporary philosophical investigations into 'language', 'action' and 'narrative'. He holds that the final stage of a phenomenology of the person would describe the 'responsible person' as the one constituted by three characteristics. Firstly, a desire for an accomplished life expressed in *self-esteem*. Secondly, a desire for an accomplished life for, and with, others expressed in *solicitude*. Thirdly, a desire for an accomplished life for, and with, others in just institutions expressed in *distributive justice*.

This is not the place to fully elaborate Ricoeur's notion of personalism, nor to show its possible application to personalist medical ethics. Still, the point I want to make is that any personalism missing such substratum and roots in philosophy, runs the danger of facile applications. It is, once again, the story of the master key and the mastermind.

In conclusion

Personalism based on the integral and adequate consideration of the person was, for Louis Janssens, not in contradiction with the foundations of traditional moral theology. His profound knowledge of the theology of Thomas Aquinas, but also his keen eye for evolution and the signs of the times enabled him to offer insights that could save magisterial teachings on sexuality and reproduction from petrifying. Thus, he successfully contributed to the declarations of the Second Vatican Council.

However, two dimensions of the person brought his thinking to the edge of traditional moral theology, even to contradict edicts of Roman theology. These dimensions are corporality and historicity. They provided a framework of thinking for the dynamic development, the growth and process of persons throughout their whole life.

It remains difficult to decide whether he had a fully fledged theory, an anthropology or a system that was phenomenological and normative. Probably, for him, personalist ethics was all of those. As for the mantra of the eight dimensions, they offer a safe guidance, provided they are called upon comprehensively, exhaustively, and above all consistently. Meanwhile, theory building has to be pursued. The interface with biomedical issues will remain the testing ground for personalist theory to prove its usefulness. The next section will, therefore, focus on the application of personalist ethics on questions of reproductive medicine.

References

1. Janssens L., Personalisme en democratisering, Brussel, Arbeiderspers, 1957.
2. Burggraeve R., The holistic personalism of Professor Magister Louis Janssens. In: Louvain Studies 27 (2002) 29-38.
3. Janssens L., Kunstmatige inseminatie: ethische beschouwingen. In: Verpleegkundigen en gemeenschapszorg 35 (1979) 220-240, [Also in English: Artificial insemination: ethical considerations. In: Louvain Studies 8 (1980-1981) 3-29].
4. Janssens L., L'inhibition de l'ovulation est-elle moralement licite? In: Ephemerides Theologicae Lovanienses 34 (1958) 357-360.
5. Janssens L., Considerations on Humanae vitae. In: Louvain Studies 2 (1968-1969) 231-253.
6. Janssens L., Moral problems involved in responsible parenthood. In: Louvain Studies 1 (1966-1967) 3-18.
7. Janssens L., Particular goods and personalist morals. In: Ethical Perspectives 6 (1999) 55-59.
8. Christie D. L., Adequately considered. An American perspective on Louis Janssens' personalist morals. Leuven, Peeters Press, 1990.
9. Selling J.A., Is a personalist ethic necessarily anthropocentric? In: Ethical Perspectives (1999) 60-66.
10. Selling J.A., The human person; In Bernard Hoose (ed.) Christian Ethics: An introduction. London, Cassell, 1998, 95-109.
11. Jans J., The foundations of an ethics of responsibility. Ethical Perspectives 3 (1996) 148-156.
12. Selling J.A., The instruction of the respect for life: I. The fundamental methodology. In: Louvain Studies 12 (1987) 212-244..
13. Grabowski J.S., Person or nature? Rival personalisms in 20th century Catholic sexual ethics. In: Studia Moralia 35 (1997) 283-312.
14. McCormick R.A., Notes on moral theology 1981-1984. In Theological Studies 10 (1990) 3-24.
15. McCormick R.A., The critical calling, Washington. DC, Georgetown University Press, 1989.

16. Johnstone B.V., The revisionist project in Roman Catholic Moral Theology. In: Studies in Christian Ethics 5 (1992) nr. 2, 18-31.
17. Selling J.A., Personalist Morals. Essays in honor of Professor Louis Janssens. Leuven, Peeters University Press, 1988.
18. Selling J.A., Proportionate reasoning and the concept of ontic evil: The moral theological legacy of Louis Janssens. In: Louvain Studies 27 (2002) 3-28.
19. Janssens L., Ontic evil and moral evil. In: Louvain Studies 4 (1972-1973) 116-156.
20. Johnstone B.V., From Physicalism to Personalism. In: Studia Moralia 30 (1990) 71-96.
21. Schotsmans P., Personalism in medical ethics. In: Ethical Perspectives 6 (1999) 10-19.
22. Schotsmans P., In vitro fertilization: the ethics of illicitness? A personalist Catholic approach. In The European Journal of Obstetrics & Gynecology and Reprodutive Biology 81 (1998) 235-241.
23. Ricoeur P., Approches de la personne. In: Esprit 57 (1990) 115-130. [Also in English: Approaching the human person. In Ethical Perspectives 6 (1999) 45-54].

27. Personalist ethics applied to reproductive medicine

Maurice De Wachter

In the previous section I briefly outlined the theory of personalist ethics at the Catholic University of Leuven beginning in the middle of the twentieth century. In a complementary way this section explores some applications of personalist ethics to reproductive medicine. They illustrate the positions held by individual authors but also by institutions such as ethics committees, counseling teams, the Faculty of Medicine and academic authorities. As in the previous section on the theory of personalist medical ethics, it is Magister Louis Janssens himself who sets the tone in a masterly article of 1979 on ethical considerations about artificial insemination, a form of assisted reproductive medicine which had been around at the Catholic University of Leuven for almost a decade[1]. Abortion, in vitro fertilization, and fetal surgery offer other examples. The latest issues on human stem cell research are momentarily still under debate, and do not yet allow one to draw a clear picture of the way personalist ethics handles them.

Abortion

During the early 1970s, Belgian society was in turmoil over the dilemma of abortion. Bills in favor were being prepared and answers from mainly religious sides were promptly issued. The debate revealed a change in the moral evaluation of the conflict between the mother's life and fetal life. Traditionally, medical indications, for instance cases of ectopic pregnancy or of uterine carcinoma, were considered by many as a justification for abortion. The reasoning went like this: because of the tension between 'being and being', a conflict may arise where either two lives will be lost, or where one is saved at the price of the other. Moreover, this practice was called 'indirect killing' because the pregnancy was terminated as a consequence of the life-saving treatment of the mother. During the 1970s, though, the conflict came to be perceived in terms of 'well-being versus being'. Some audiences found it difficult to accept this widening of the medical indication for abortion into psychological and social indications. Yet, Louis Janssens told me that he believed that the psychic destruction of a woman was worse than to take the physical life of a fetus[2]. He would also discuss these issues with graduate students in his courses and seminars. Course notes of 1973 show how he proceeded with caution. He began by pointing out that classical moral theology never rejected abortion absolutely, witness the notion of 'indirect abortion'. He then wondered whether the presence of a fetus could ever constitute a serious danger for a meaningful bodily existence of the pregnant woman. And if so, would that justify an interruption of the pregnancy? Despite his belief in our duty to give the fetus a chance to live, Janssens thought that this conflict may become inhuman. The various answers given – from rejection of abortion, to acceptance of strictly medical indications, to acceptance in cases of rape or serious deformity – all boiled down to two fundamentally different points of departure: one where the value of the fetus prevails, the other where the mother's interests prevail. While acknowledging the usefulness of the first opinion as a remedy against bias or exaggerated certainty of one's viewpoint, Janssens chose the second position.

During the late 1980s and early 1990s the Leuven Commission for Medical Ethics issued several position papers and advisory documents concerning the Belgian bills on abortion[3]. In each of them the connection with personalism is made explicit, for instance when talking about our duties to respect unborn human life, it is said that 'in order to approach this problem, the best we can do is to start from the necessary respect for the human person, considered in all his dimensions and relations'[3].

Artificial insemination and the role of a counseling team

The first artificial insemination with donor semen (AID) at the K.U.Leuven took place in August 1971. By 1982 a total of 674 couples had been treated, resulting in 509 pregnancies. Particular to the service was the presence of a counseling team consisting of several gynecologists and obstetricians, an andrologist, a urologist, a psychiatrist, and an ethicist. Opinions were constantly under revision. A few members were of the opinion that AID had been accepted in our society as a possible solution for undesired childlessness which has its cause in the husband. Others made reservations, admitting only cases with absolute and definitive male sterility or genetic defects in the husband. Rhesus incompatibility and proven immunization were also acceptable indications. Finally, functional sterility of the couple as a whole was recognized. By 1975 the team issued its mission statement as follows:

> In well-defined cases of undesired childlessness where, after serious investigation, after serene deliberation and a mature choice, and where the possibility exists to offer a higher level of quality of life as well as of fulfillment of life, we deem it ethically acceptable to apply the treatment of AID with utter care and a sense of responsibility[4].

In the same year of 1975 the Leuven Commission for Medical Ethics was installed. Artificial insemination by donor was the very first topic to be addressed and approved. It was known that Janssens and several of his colleagues (Jos Ghoos, Pierre De Locht, Maurice De Wachter) were directly or indirectly involved in the clinical counseling team of the AID program. The first advice of the ethics committee reflects and approves the progressive viewpoints of these people. A more detailed description of this advice was given above (see Chapter VI, 19). This document is a precursor of Janssens' article of 1979.

During that same decade Janssens brought his 'ethics of responsibility based upon the person' to bear on the practice of artificial insemination. The result was his *'magnum opus'*, the prestigious article of 1979[1]. The article is not only logically clear, and illustrative of the progressive complexities in ethical reasoning, but also entices those involved to proceed with caution. For both homologous (AIH) and heterologous or donor (AID) insemination he considered the well-being of the couple, of the child, and of society. For homologous insemination (AIH) he first justified in vivo practices, then in vitro. About heterologous insemination he, for obvious reasons, mentions in vitro practice only. In short, the article displays an accomplished skill of fine-tuning in ethical considerations.

For homologous in vitro insemination, recently illustrated by the birth of Louise Brown, Janssens saw three major moral aspects that deserved attention. Firstly came safety and success rates; secondly, somatic and psychic integrity of the child; thirdly, the destruction of spare embryos. Safety and success, he said, were primarily the responsibility of scientists, but nonetheless of major interest to the moralist. Indeed, he could never approve of mere experimentation with human life for the sake of progress. The child's integrity was another aspect to be tested by scientists, but again of great ethical relevance since the person is a subject in corporality. Finally, regarding the destruction of supernumerary embryos, Janssens was rather skeptical of Steptoe's opinion that in natural procreation also many fertilized eggs are lost. He found this argument too physicalistic, and too weak to justify a responsible choice[1].

Regarding heterologous in vitro insemination Janssens insisted on the welfare of the child which would only be warranted if parents, over and above accepting their biological sterility, were capable of psychological parenthood. For Janssens this condition was essential and decisive in the admission of the couple to fertility treatment.

Noteworthy is Janssens' skepticism about the then quite common practice of never telling the child about the way it was conceived. Instead, he thought it wise to act according to the psychological capacity of the child and according to circumstances. Donors, he thought, should also remain anonymous. The practice of asking only married men to donate was a practice of which he approved.

Finally, with regard to the social impact of AID, Janssens restated one last time his personalist answer: 'The moral question is about reasons (*ratio proportionata*) that would justify fertility treatment, and whether according to rules of priority what will be realized outweighs the negative aspects.'[1] Once the emotional opposition to AID has been cleared, we should be able to draw the lessons from experience and determine whether or not the practice is respectful of human dignity of the person considered fully in himself/herself and in his/her relations. 'It is my humble opinion that these experiences converge, such that ethics must not radically condemn, rather it must emphasize the delicate matter at stake, where a critical selection of both couples and donors is demanded'[1].

Ten years later, enriched by more experience and alerted by some fundamental objections, the Leuven Commission on Medical Ethics issued a second advice on AID (1989)[3]. In it, the Commission addressed the question of whether AID was acceptable in principle. The major obstacle remained of the introduction of a third party into the intimacy of the marital relationship. Nevertheless, most members of the Commission were of the opinion that the final decision should be left with the conscience of the fully informed couple, provided there were good reasons to expect that the marital relationship would be improved by this procedure. However, mention was made of the fact that Leuven with its AID program was isolated from the other Catholic universities. (For more details see Chapter IX, 19.)

After another ten years, in 1998, the question about AID's acceptability in principle was still on the agenda of the Commission. Its third advice on AID confirmed the previous division of opinion but insisted on the necessity of a decision to be taken by the Academic Authority in the matter. (See Chapter VI, 20.)

A characteristic quality of Janssens' personalism is its openness to other disciplines and tolerance of other people's opinion. Both qualities appear repeatedly in the 1979 article on artificial insemination. In the introduction Janssens writes that a difference of moral opinion may "depend on the measure in which people count with the facts of science, but also on the foundations upon which they have built their ethics or on the way they approach problems"[1]. A particular instance of such difference of opinion is directly linked to this article. We saw that Janssens pleaded for acceptance of AIH and, under certain conditions, for AID. On the other hand, the well-known American theologian Richard McCormick, who was a fervent admirer of Janssens' explanations of the criterion of the human person integrally and adequately considered[5], while also accepting AIH, disagreed on AID[6]. Here is a brief description of what I have explained at some length elsewhere[7].

McCormick, as a member of the Ethics Committee of the American Fertility Society, pointed out that the personalist criterion demands careful handling in the area of sexual ethics, where humans are always 'liable to self-interested judgments and insensitivity to the call of basic values'[5]. In the opening passage of the 'General considerations' of the report McCormick argued that personalism may contain 'a moral ambiguity and pluralism (which) calls for openness, caution and willingness to revise evaluations'[8]. Further down he stated that "what is promotive or detrimental to the person cannot be assessed solely in terms of individual impact but must take into account overall social impact as well"[8]. When the Ethics Committee accepted both AIH and AID, McCormick wrote an Appendix called 'Dissent on the use of third parties', that is, sperm donors, ovum donors, or surrogate womb. Listing five points, McCormick remarked that AID severs procreation from the marital union, compromises the child's self-identity, might multiply adulteries, is a move towards eugenics, and tends to absolutize sterility as a disvalue. He concluded that AID is 'not for the good of persons integrally and adequately considered. It involves risks to basic dimensions of our flourishing. Such risks to basic values outweigh, in a prudential calculus, individual procreative desires or needs. In summary: when calculus involves individual benefit versus institutional risk of harm, the latter should take precedence'[8]. Obviously, for some, the benefit of the single person or couple will be dominant, for others, the potential risk to society takes precedence over individual benefits. It is worth noting that Janssens said exactly that in 1979: "From a personalist standpoint what must be examined is what the intervention as a whole means for the promotion of the human persons who are involved and for their relationships"[1]. To the best of my knowledge, both Jansens and McCormick had no difficulty respecting each other's opinion. The question must be asked, however, if we are faced here with a possible weakness in the system, due to equivocal applications of the eight dimensions.

In vitro fertilization

New medical technologies such as in vitro fertilization (IVF) often mean serious challenges to traditional ethics. Here, the personalist approach may offer an ethical frame for their integration. Thus, for Paul Schotsmans, IVF can be ethically integrated provided the following three conditions are met: a stable marital relation caring for a child; a minimal protection of the embryo; and society's quality control of the technique in a democratic society[9].

Firstly, recent developments in sexual ethics allow us to see IVF not as a substitution for sexual intimacy, but rather as its prolongation[10]. Here, the criterion of the relation becomes a creative principle for ordering the recreative, procreative and institutional dimensions of human sexuality. 'For all these reasons, Schotsmans says, the ethical requirement of a stable, heterosexual couple becomes an urgent clinical necessity'[10]. Indeed, children need parents, not just procreators. And only good marital partners make good parents. Clinically, this criterion may be met by adequate counseling in the medical fertility team. Visibly, this approach is very much in line with Janssens' requirement that the parents, having mourned the loss of biological parenthood, be capable of psychological parenthood. For Janssens this requirement was a *sine qua non*.

Secondly, because the human embryo is our equal, because the human zygote is carrier of possible poles of reciprocity, we can never dispose of it. 'The willingness to dispose of the human embryo is equivalent to giving in to the temptation to decide who may be our equals'. After all, this is a question of ontological solidarity amongst humans, which we must always confirm, never contradict.

Thirdly comes the regulatory side. IVF clinics need to develop quality control. Couples in treatment should be informed, and remain free to exit the course of treatment at any time. Meanwhile, society ought to develop guidelines for fertility centers. Democratic states must not leave the development of these techniques open to arbitrary initiatives, as is unfortunately still the case in Belgium.

With the conclusion that IVF can be ethically integrated, Schotsmans, obviously, begs to differ from the position taken by Roman Congregation for the doctrine of faith in its 1987 Instruction. He offers three arguments. Firstly, the Instruction reduces marriage to bodily union only. Secondly, it considers illicit every act that does not reach the fullness of its meaning (it calls homologous IVF illicit in itself). Thirdly, it ignores the possible conflict between unitive and procreative dimensions.

Obviously, this personalist approach offered by Schotsmans takes into account the various advisory documents on IVF-ET issued by the Leuven Commission on Medical Ethics starting in 1984 through 1989[3]. These documents are explicitly described in Chapter VI, 22.

Fetal surgery

Fetal surgery in cases of twin-to-twin transfusion syndrome, that is where one twin is transfusing the other thereby threatening the life of both, is life threatening. In Chapter VII, 25 and X, 37 the underlying ethical dilemma is identified as 'a conflict between the mother's well-being and the well-being of the fetus, or, as in the case of a multiple pregnancy, between the well-being of a healthy and a diseased fetus.' Starting in 1994, therapy by fetoscopic cord ligations was performed at the K.U.Leuven, with informed consent given by the parents and after approval by the local ad hoc ethics committee of the University Hospitals. Later the K.U.Leuven ethics committee offered principles and advice on the matter of prenatal diagnosis. In 2001, the Committee concluded that the correct doctor-patient relationship should be neither determined by paternalism nor by extreme patient autonomy. Instead, it ought to be a collaborating relationship, open and transparent, in mutual respect. The Committee, in the same advice of 2001 regarding prenatal diagnosis, mentioned three instances of possible 'slippery slope' effects, should the parents request that the pregnancy be terminated. Firstly, aborting handicapped fetuses may lead to active euthanasia of handicapped newborn babies. Secondly, given the absence of clear differentiation between light, moderate, severe and extreme handicaps, the decision may be taken arbitrarily. Thirdly, society may become more intolerant of handicapped people, and blame parents for not having prevented them from being born. Regarding the interruption of pregnancy, the Committee states that the parental decision is 'to be respected, although it may be questioned.'

In its rationale, the Committee quotes the papal encyclical *Evangelium vitae* (1995) where Pope John Paul II addressed women who had had an abortion[11]. To those women he said that 'certainly, what happened was and remains terribly wrong. But do not give in to discouragement and do not lose hope ... The father of mercies is ready to give you his forgiveness' (John Paul II, 99). The Ethics committee interprets this passage as 'profound pastoral understanding' which 'signifies that abortion remains ethically evil but, in the tragic confrontation of the human being with suffering and shortcomings, it can be an acceptable evil and an ethically justifiable choice in conscience. Therefore, it follows that in all openness and transparency, the conscientious choice made by the patient should be respected and surrounded with the greatest care.' One wonders how likely it is that this is what the Pope meant. On the other hand, the Ethics committee, in its courageous effort to promote an open, humane and creative support system for spouses caught in such terrible dilemmas, offers several proposals, principles and further advice, all of which deserve to be commended. For the detail of those points I refer again to Chapter VII, 25. My reservation is strictly and only about the interpretation of the encyclical given by the Committee. My reason for the reservation lies in Louis Janssens' aversion of the distinction between the moral and the pastoral. This distinction was foreign to him. Janssens 'never opted to use the traditional distinction between 'objective' and 'subjective' as a general methodological principle of interpretation of human behavior.'[12] It leads to 'deculpabilization' at the subjective level, but runs the risk of 'infantilization'. This means, for instance, that 'a decision about birth control that is not in line with official teaching is necessarily regarded as ethically inferior, while it may well have been the fruit of deliberate and conscious choice'[12]. One must fear that the Ethics committee chose at the same time for 'Roman theology' and for personalist ethics. In doing so, it may have maneuvered itself into an awkward position. Remember, you can't have your cake and eat it too! But, then, fetal surgery undoubtedly will offer new opportunities to rethink and, if needed, revise earlier statements of the Ethics Committee. It did so in the past, and deserves to be commended for doing so.

In conclusion

One could say, in all fairness, that the personalist ethics of responsibility enabled Janssens to address all delicate situations he encountered in medicine during his long career as a moral theologian. If it is true that he wanted to save the magisterial teaching of the Church from petrifying, it is equally true that he wanted to save concrete people from being hurt.

Janssens was open to insights coming from the humanities and the life sciences that would help to solve problems of human suffering. He trusted their results when he was convinced that they showed a promotion of humanness for persons. The last footnote of his article on artificial insemination is revealing in this sense. The note is about 'serious research' proving that, after responsible selection, the experience of people treated by heterologous insemination shows that positive aspects outweigh the lack of biological parenthood. On the other hand, when scientists were not able to convince him, he would ask a few simple questions, the answer to which could not possibly be given by science at that point in time. For instance, and again in the same article on artificial insemination, he questioned the then commonly accepted practice of secrecy towards the child. He (innocently) asked if we really knew that telling the child about the way it was conceived would always be harmful. How prophetic! We now know that telling the child is rarely harmful, whereas not telling has caused serious harm. This may be a last example of how Louis Janssens was able to strike a balance between converging positive experiences on the one hand and a critical consideration in light of the personalist criterion: the person adequately considered in himself/herself and his/her relations. The outcome of which was what he called 'my humble opinion'[3].

References

1. Janssens L., Kunstmatige inseminatie: ethische beschouwingen. In: Verpleegkundigen en gemeenschapszorg 35 (1979) 220-240, [Also in English: Artificial insemination: ethical considerations. In: Louvain Studies 8 (1980-1981) 3-29].
2. De Wachter M.A.M., Abortus als ethisch dilemma. Leuven/Lochem, Acco/De Tijdstroom, 1974.
3. Vermylen J. and P. Schotsmans (ed.), Ethiek in de kliniek, Leuven, Universitaire Pers, 2000.
4. De Wachter M.A.M., I. Brosens, P. Nijs, O. Steeno, A. Van Assche, R. Vereecken, Menselijke vruchtbaarheid en geboortenplanning. Brussel, Elsevier Sequoia, 1976.
5. McCormick R.A., The critical calling, Washington. DC, Georgetown University Press, 1989.
6. McCormick R.A., Notes on moral theology 1981-1984. In Theological Studies 10 (1990) 3-24.
7. De Wachter M.A.M., How useful is Leuven personalism in the world of bioethics? The test case of artificial insemination. In European Journal of Obstetrics & Gynecology and Reproductive Biology 81 (1998) 227-233.
8. American Fertility Society. Ethical considerations of the new reproductive technologies. In Fertility and Sterility 53 (1990) (Suppl. 2) 1-109.
9. Schotsmans P., Personalism in medical ethics. In: Ethical Perspectives 6 (1999) 10-19.

10. Schotsmans P., In vitro fertilization: the ethics of illicitness? A personalist Catholic approach. In The European Journal of Obstetrics & Gynecology and Reproductive Biology 81 (1998) 235-241.
11. John Paul II, Evangelium vitae, Rome, Libreria Editrice Vaticana, 1995.
12. Burggraeve R., The holistic personalism of Professor Magister Louis Janssens. In Louvain Studies 27 (2002) 29-38.

28. Memoirs of a dialogue

Based on interviews with Marcel Renaer

In 1962, Jacques Ferin, Professor of Medical Gynecology at the Catholic University of Leuven, published in the *Acta Endocrinologica* an article entitled "Artificial induction of hypo-estrogenic amenorrhea with methylestrenolone, or with lynestrenol". This article, which proved that the continuous intake of a progestogen pill could suppress menstruation and induce amenorrhea, came to the attention of Louis Janssens, professor at the Faculty of Theology. He argued in November 1963 in *Ephemerides Theologicae Lovanienses* that "salve mejore judicio" such hormonal therapy would be morally acceptable in some cases to avoid pregnancy. The view of Louis Janssens expressed in his article was the start of much discussion amongst theologians. While some agreed and others disagreed, there were also Catholic theologians and philosophers who changed their opinion continuously. It was said that the influential Monseigneur Heylen was for on even days and against on odd days.

During this period the obstetrician professor, JA Schockaert, started "Les Journées Louvanistes sur la Sexualité". These were regular weekend meetings at his home with the international participation of gynecologists, theologians, philosophers and people from other disciplines. At that time Cardinal Suenens defended strongly the official view of the Church and was opposed to the use of the pill for temporary contraception, as well as against tubal sterilization for permanent contraception. When, at a meeting, a German gynecologist asked "Warum?" (Why?) he replied: "Was Rome sagt" (It is what Rome says). Some came like the American Jesuit John Ford to defend the very conservative attitude. These meetings led to the foundation of the Institute for Family and Sexuality Sciences at the K.U.Leuven. At this multidisciplinary school students could follow a two-year course to obtain a degree of licenciate in Family and Sexuality Sciences.

The initial position of many leading international Catholics in the field was also against the use of the pill for birth control. However, people like André Hellegers, Joseph Fuchs and Cardinal Suenens changed their position over time and accepted the use of the pill for contraception within marriage. The opposition by Catholic leaders is illustrated by the following incident. In 1963, Marcel Renaer, Professor of Obstetrics and Gynecology and also Professor of Medical Ethics, was invited by John McClure Brown, professor of Obstetrics and Gynaecology at the Hammersmith Hospital, to come to London and briefly address a meeting on contraception at the Royal College of Obstetricians and Gynaecologists. He knew that Renaer had a different view the leading British Catholics and Renaer was given four minutes to make his presentation. The British Catholic view was presented at the meeting by a professor of neurology at a London medical school. Renaer had his presentation the evening before corrected by a friend, Geoffrey Dixon, gynecologist at the Hammersmith Hospital. In his short presentation he said:

> it is well known that Roman Catholics are against, but I shall add that there are a few important Catholics, such as professor magister Louis Janssens at the Catholic University in Leuven and John F Kennedy, President of the United States, who are prepared to allow for exceptions.

The neurologist, who made a long speech to defend the Catholic position and to condemn the use of the pill, followed his brief presentation. He told the audience that the documents of the Church teachings are based on the necessity of having children and this is what sexual intercourse is for. The audience was apparently uninterested in his argumentation. After the meeting the neurologist congratulated Renaer for his very good English. The end of the story is that, in 2002, an article appeared in the international Catholic journal *The Tablet* on marriage morals from the same professor of neurology in which he admitted that he had committed an error and that his argumentation had been incomplete. The error was that sexuality in marriage is not only for reproduction, but also for mutual comfort.

The Second Vatican Council was opened in 1962 and Suenens was one of the four cardinals to lead the discussions. Suenens was very concerned with being informed about gynecological practices and frequently attended the weekly staff meetings at the office of a gynecologist in Brussels in order to follow the discussions of clinical cases. By the time Johannes XXIII died, in 1963, Suenens had changed progressively and no longer had objections against the use of the pill for family planning. One evening, upon his return from Rome, when he had just bought a little car, Suenens came to the home of Professor Renaer. He recounted how, in the middle of the council meeting with 2500 bishops (most of them being of a curial opinion and some of a more liberal opinion), he told the audience of bishops " Please, let us not have a second Galileo Gallilei incident!" Gallilei was condemned by the "infallible" church leaders of his day for his heretical teachings about the earth's rotation around the sun. Suenens, as a good friend, advised Monsignor Montini, the new pope Paulus VI, to rewrite and modernize the encyclical *Casti Connubii* (published in 1931) in order to allow the use of the pill.

Cardinal Suenens is reported to have asked Pope Paulus VI three times to rewrite *Casti Connubii*: why should a woman with three or four children not be allowed to take the pill? The Pope replied that he was not going to do so because he did not want to enter history as the pope who had given permission to avoid pregnancy with the pill.

In the 1960s, there was great malaise over family planning amongst practicing Catholics in Belgium, particularly in Flanders. It was well known that the pill was prescribed for contraception at the Catholic University in Leuven. A short story illustrates the confusion amongst the people. Traditionally Marcel Renaer took a break with his family during the Easter holiday on the Belgian coast in the small village of Wenduine. Each year around Easter the curate had to read the annual briefing on marriage duties, which stressed the duty of having children. No method was allowed to be used that could limit procreation, the core duty of marriage. During his Easter holiday in 1963 the curate took the opportunity to come and see Renaer for more clarification:

> Professor, it is Easter again. It is going to happen again. Our good Christians are coming for confession again: 65% of them come to confess that they have been using coitus interruptus. This is all that Easter confession is about! This makes Easter for me the unhappiest time of the year. Please, how can you allow the pill at the Catholic University of Leuven? Please explain to us!

Great efforts were taken by a group of prominent Belgian Catholics to convince the bishops in Rome to review the encyclical *Casti*

Connubii. On two occasions the group drafted an open letter. The letter was translated into several languages and a small group of Flemish Catholic activists traveled to Rome to distribute the open letter, with the help of young Scheut missionaries in training in Rome, amongst the 2500 bishops. Although many bishops were in favor of change, the new encyclical *Humanae vitae* in 1968 confirmed the previous position of the church.

In 1970, Professor Louis Janssens published, in the Catholic journal *Pastor Bonus*, a critical article on *Humanae vitae*. He argued, apparently with the consent of Cardinal Suenens, that between the years '68 and '70 a number of statements were incorrect. One of them was that *Humanae vitae* was not an "infallible" document and that the conditions for infallibility were not fulfilled. Not many colleagues of Louis Janssens have reacted against *Humanae vitae*. Louis Janssens died at the age of 94 in 2003. He was one of the few famous theologians who never became a Monsignor.

PART 3

REPRODUCTIVE MEDICINE AT CATHOLIC UNIVERSITIES AROUND THE WORLD

CHAPTER IX

FERTILITY SERVICES AND CLINICAL RESEARCH

Beginning as early as the late Middle Agess, the Catholic Church established an impressive number of Catholic universities world-wide. Within these, many have a school of Medicine: four in Europe, two in the Far East, two in South America and three in the United States. The list may not be exhaustive, but it includes most, if not all, major Catholic schools of medicine in the world.

Europe:

- Università Cattolica del Sacro Cuore, Rome, Italy
- Katholieke Universiteit Leuven (K.U. Leuven), Belgium
- Université Catholique de Louvain (U.C.L), Belgium
- Radboud Universiteit Nijmegen, The Netherlands

Far East:

- University of Santo Tomas, Manila, Philippines
- Catholic University of Daegu, Daegu, South Korea

South America:

- Universidad Católica de Córdoba, Córdoba, Argentina
- Pontificia Universidad Católica de Chile, Santiago, Chile

USA:

- Georgetown University, Washington DC
- Loyola University, Chicago, Michigan
- Saint Louis University, St Louis, Missouri

In this chapter we report on our investigation of the clinical services in fertility and sterility and the research activities in reproductive medicine at these medical schools.

29. Fertility services

In 2004, the Head of the Department of Obstetrics and Gynecology or the Director of Reproductive Medicine at eleven of the twelve above mentioned university hospitals were each sent a questionnaire in order to obtain information about the clinical practice of reproductive medicine at their hospital. The questionnaire concerned the clinical services for contraception, abortion and infertility.

It was clear from the beginning that several university hospitals were not going to be forthcoming with information. At some places the University Authority was withholding information; in others, the management were unwilling to communicate the information. In all these cases, staff members were identified who were knowledgeable regarding the clinical practice of reproductive medicine at the university hospital and who were willing to supply the information. All this information must therefore be considered as first-hand information. No direct information was obtained from the Catholic University of Daegu in South Korea.

In addition, the mission statements and the clinical services that are offered at the university hospitals in the field of reproductive medicine were investigated via the websites of each university and their university hospital.

After a brief history and the official mission statement of each of the Catholic universities a summary is presented of the fertility services at the university hospitals.

1. Università Cattolica del Sacro Cuore, Rome, Italy

History

The Università Cattolica del Sacro Cuore was officially inaugurated in 1921. Today, fourteen programs, home to over 40,000 students, are distributed throughout the Milan, Rome, Brescia, Piacenza and Campobasso campuses.

In 1958, the official decree for the opening of a medical school in Rome was approved and the Biological Institutes and the Policlinic were finally built in Rome, the latter bearing the name of Father A. Gemelli. The medical school was built in the vast, beautiful property located on the top of Monte Mario, the highest hill of the city's northwestern side, overlooking the Vatican. In 1961, Pope John XXIII solemnized the birth of the medical school, with the first medical doctors graduating in 1967. The school now offers both medical and dentistry programs.

Mission statement

The Università Cattolica is an academic community designed to contribute to the development of specified studies, scientific research, and the preparation of young adults for work and service in research, teaching, and work in public and private professional fields. The Università Cattolica approaches this goal through a superior academic education, joined with the basic principles of Christianity.

Taking the Catholic name and exhibiting faithfulness to the Church represent an inalienable opportunity for the Università del Sacro Cuore to approach research and teaching in all fields of knowledge, and in particular the quintessential questions of our time, with scientific rigor and the necessary intellectual openness.

Fertility services

The information on fertility services was obtained from a senior staff member of the Department of Obstetrics and Gynecology.

- The medical school in Rome follows the teaching of the Catholic Church in matters relating to human reproduction" (Table 29.1).
- Condoms and oral contraceptives are not prescribed because they separate the unitive from the procreative meaning of the sexual act.
- The intrauterine contraceptive device and emergency contraception are not prescribes, since they are seen as preventing implantation and, therefore, as causing an early abortion.

Research in infertility has focussed for many years on reconstructive tubo-ovarian surgery. However, in vitro fertilization in patients with irreparable tubal damage is not performed. The technique of gametes intratubal transfer (GIFT) is considered ethically acceptable and therefore practiced.

2. Katholieke Universiteit Leuven (K.U.Leuven), Belgium

History

Founded in 1425 by Pope Martin V, the Catholic University of Leuven/Louvain bears the honor of being the oldest Catholic university in the world still in existence and the oldest university in the Low

Table 29.1. Clinical services in reproductive medicine at universities strictly following the Church directives

Contraception
– natural methods	yes
– condom	no
– pill	no
– IUCD	no
– emergency pill	no

Sterilization
– on demand	no
– medical	no

Abortion
– on demand	no
– socio-economic	no
– medical	no
– life-threatening condition	no

Donor insemination
– married couple	no
– unmarried couple	no
– single	no
– lesbian	no

Reproductive surgery yes

In vitro fertilization
– married couple	no
– unmarried	no
– single	no
– lesbian	no
– egg donation	no

Countries. In its early days this university was modeled on the universities of Paris, Cologne and Vienna. In a short time it grew into one of the largest and most renowned universities in Europe.

When it was founded, the University had three faculties: law, medicine and the arts. Its first teachers came from Paris and Cologne. The Faculty of Theology was added in 1432.

The theologian and humanist, Erasmus, the geographer, Mercator, and the anatomist, Vesalius, frequented the University in the sixteenth century. Louvain attracted students from the four corners of Europe and became one of the foremost universities of the time.

The university's fortunes have followed the ups and downs of history: it was closed under French domination (1797), re-opened by the bishops in 1834, and bombed in the two world wars (losing its entire library in the fire of 1914).

The university is located in Flanders, the Dutch-speaking northern part of Belgium. With the Dutch language's steady rise to renewed prominence, the university was eventually split in 1968 into two independent universities. The French-speaking Université Catholique de Louvain (U.C.L.) moved, in 1971, to the newly-built campus in Louvain-la-Neuve. The Dutch-speaking Katholieke Universiteit Leuven (K.U.Leuven) remained in the historic town of Leuven.

The **K.U.Leuven**, the Flemish university of Catholic signature, has the legal statute of a private institution.

Mission statement

As a university it is an academic institution where research that opens up new horizons and knowledge transfer are both essential and complementary.

As a university it distinguishes itself from other research centers by its autonomous statement of problems, by the disinterested character of its fundamental research, by its focus on education and by the fact that within its walls it encompasses almost all academic disciplines.

As a university it distinguishes itself from other educational institutions by the fact that its teaching is based on and nourished by its own research and by its interdisciplinary approach.

It defines its tasks and priorities autonomously, and the members of its academic staff enjoy academic freedom in the exercise of their duties.

In the acquisition of knowledge the K.U.Leuven is guided only by the requirements of research methodology and deontology.

In a number of fields the university aspires to a place among the centers of excellence in Europe and in the world.

As a Catholic university, the K.U.Leuven is a critical center of thought within the Catholic community, and as such it is deeply concerned with the relationship between science and faith, and with the dialogue between church and the world.

On the basis of its Christian view of man and society, the K.U.Leuven reflects on the axiological, ethical and religious problems emerging from developments in science and technology, and from changes in social and cultural life. This reflection takes place in a free and open climate, and in collaboration with kindred universities. Special attention is paid to the personal dignity of human beings, to the protection of the weak, and to justice and peace. The

K.U.Leuven also creates a spiritual climate which favors the full human and religious development of the members of the university community.

Fertility services

Table 29.2 summarizes the clinical services in reproductive medicine at the Gasthuisberg Hospital of the K.U.Leuven.

Table 29.2. Fertility Services at Catholic university hospitals in the Low Countries

	K.U.Leuven	U.C.L.	St Radboud
Contraception			
– natural family planning	yes	yes	yes
– condom	yes	yes	yes
– pill	yes	yes	yes
– IUCD	yes	yes	yes
– emergency pill	yes	yes	yes
Sterilization			
– on demand	yes	yes	yes
– medical	yes	yes	yes
Abortion			
– on demand	no	no	no
– socio-economic	no	no	no
– medical indication	yes	yes	yes
– life-threatening condition	yes	yes	yes
Donor insemination			
– married couple	yes	no	no
– unmarried couple	yes	no	no
– single	no	no	no
– lesbian	no	no	no
Reproductive surgery	yes	yes	yes
In vitro fertilization			
– married couple	yes	yes	yes
– unmarried couple	yes	yes	yes
– single	no	no	no
– lesbian	no	no	no
Egg donation	yes	no	no
Embryo cryopreservation	yes	yes	yes

3. Université Catholique de Louvain (U.C.L.), Belgium

After the split in 1971, the Université Catholique de Louvain was established in Louvain-la-Neuve, a town created south of Brussels for that purpose. It was comprised of a new university campus and, in Brussels, a new Catholic university hospital, St Luc.

Mission statement

For all of six centuries, the Université Catholique de Louvain (U.C.L.) has been dedicated to acquiring knowledge and passing it on from generation to generation for the greater good of society.

Whether in our western countries with their heavy demands for quality health care, or in the countries of the southern hemisphere, society has an ever greater need for people who are able to care for their fellow human beings. We need not just general practitioners and specialists, surgeons, pharmacists and dentists, but also people trained in hospital management, public health issues, preventive medicine, crisis intervention whether in the context of natural or other disasters, in urgent humanitarian aid and in many other areas.

The U.C.L. contributes to human health by training men and women in all the medical disciplines.

Fertility services

Table 29.2 summarizes the services in reproductive medicine at the University Hospital St Luc in Brussels as completed by Professor Jacques Donnez, Head of the Department of Obstetrics and Gynecology.

4. Radboud Universiteit Nijmegen, The Netherlands

History

In 1923, 27 professors, 3 assistants and 189 students started the Catholic University Nijmegen. In a number of townhouses they studied theology, the arts, philosophy and law.

The name was changed, in September 2004, into Radboud University Nijmegen. Today, the University Radboud Nijmegen and the University Medical Center (UMC) St Radboud have around 10,000 collaborators and 14,500 students.

The name Radboud University Nijmegen refers to the university's history. In 1905, the Radboud Foundation was set up to promote Catholic higher education in general, and to create a Catholic university, in particular. Thanks to the contributions of the Catholic population of the country, the Catholic university was established in 1923. The name Radboud University Nijmegen confirms this close tie with the Dutch Catholic community. The university no longer carries the name 'Catholic', but stresses its Catholic roots.

Mission statement

The logo of the UMC St Radboud Nijmegen is: *"Gedreven door kenn-nis, bewogen door mensen"("Driven by knowledge, motivated by people)".*

The University Medical Centrum St Radboud is a center of knowledge and reputable for excellence in academic medicine and medical care. Knowledge links, research, teaching and patient care are at the heart of the organization.

Fertility services

Table 29.2 summarizes the clinical services in reproductive medicine at the UMC St Radboud hospital as provided by Dr. Jan Kremer, Director of Fertility Services.

In 1987 the Commission for Medical Ethics approved the use of donor insemination as a treatment for male infertility in a married couple. The preservation of the anonymity of the donor was recommended. However, the Commission stressed the lack of accurate information on the psychological implications for the couple, the donor and the offspring and the need of follow-up of all three parties involved in order to adapt, if needed, the recommendation in the future. In 2002, the Commission for Medical Ethics extensively reviewed the practice of donor insemination and in vitro fertilization with sperm or egg donation. After careful evaluation of the arguments for and against and the potential risks for all parties involved, the commission, by a majority vote, advised against donor insemination and in vitro fertilization with sperm or egg donation. The main issue was the potential conflict of interest and whether or not sufficient data would be available to estimate the long-term effects of conception by using donor gametes for the future child. The negative advice was based on two considerations: firstly, the duty of physicians not to cause harm before fulfilling the wish of others and, secondly, the duty to protect the weak against potential harm.

5. University of Santo Tomas, Manila, Philippines

The University of Santo Tomas, founded in 1611, is the oldest existing university in Asia. It was originally conceived as a school to prepare young men for the priesthood. In 1645, Pope Innocent X elevated it to the rank of a university and in 1680 it was subsequently placed under royal patronage.

Pope Leo XIII made the University of Santo Tomas a "Pontifical University" on September 17 1902, and in 1974 Pope Pius XII bestowed upon it the title of "The Catholic University of the Philippines".

Mission statement

The University of Santo Tomas, the Pontifical and Catholic University of the Philippines under the inspiration and patronage of St. Thomas Aquinas, commits itself to the pursuit of truth and to the preservation, advancement and transmission of knowledge in the arts and sciences, both sacred and civil, through the use of reason illumined by faith.

The university affirms its role in the formation of men and women to become competent and compassionate professionals committed to the service of the Church, the nation and the global community.

Reproductive medicine

The University of Santo Tomas strictly follows the instructions of the Catholic Church (Table 29.1). The department of obstetoics and gynecology at the University of Santo Tomas Hospital promotes only the natural family methods and has no program of assisted reproductive technologies.

6. Catholic University of Daegu, South Korea

History

The history of the Catholic University of Daegu (C.U.D.) begins in 1914. Since then the university has undergone many changes. When it was first opened in 1914 it was given the name of Saint Ustino School of Theology. In 1952 the university adopted the name Hyosung Women's University. In 2000 the university adopted its current name, Catholic University of Daegu. Through all the name changes one thing has always remained constant, a commitment to education. The university has three main campuses operating under its jurisdiction: St. Ustino School of Theology in Namsan-dong, Daegu; St. Luke School of Medicine, Daemyung-hdong, Daegu; and the main campus of Hyosung located in Hayang, C.U.D. is the largest Catholic university in Korea. It has about 17,000 students. C.U.D. is founded on the principles of Christianity and defines itself and all its programs through this Christ-centered spirit.

Reproductive medicine

No direct information was obtained on the fertility services and on research in reproductive medicine at St. Luke School of Medicine.

A search on PubMed of the National Library of Medicine revealed no publications on topics in reproductive medicine, such as natural family planning, contraception, infertility, sterility and in vitro fertilization.

7. *Universidad Católica de Córdoba, Córdoba, Argentina*

History

The university was founded by a Belgian jesuit in 1955 and has had a Faculty of Medicine since 1959.

Clinical practice

Since 1999, the Catholic University of Cordoba has had its own bioethics center to provide guidance from the perspective of a catholic institution. The university strictly follows the instructions of the Church magisterium and has issued the following guidelines:

- Life must be respected without any restriction from the moment of conception to its natural ending.
- No objectives, no matter how valuable or noble, justify the means, particularly if they affect the dignity of the human person.
- The concepts of responsible parenthood and of a conscious regulation of the number of children a couple can have are valid; in this context natural family planning methods are recommended.
- It is immoral to use contraceptive methods that may potentially act as an abortive agent, such as the intrauterine device.
- Tubal sterilization is rejected as a method of contraception. This does not exclude tubal sterilization from being performed for medical reasons.
- Under no circumstances is abortion acceptable.
- All medical interventions guided to defeat sterility have to be considered in relation to a heterosexual, stable couple and in relation to the sexual act and the dignity the act demands.
- Donor insemination is not acceptable.
- In vitro fertilization is not acceptable for the previously mentioned reason. Moreover, the technique can cause destruction or damage of embryos, which is ethically not acceptable.

8. Pontificia Universidad Católica de Chile, Santiago, Chile

History

The Archbishop of Santiago founded the university in 1888 and Pope Leo XIII officially approved the university as Pontificia Universidad Católica de Chile in 1889. The university has 18 schools distributed across four campuses in Santiago and one regional campus located in southern Chile.

Approximately 20,000 students participate in its undergraduate and graduate programs, which cover a wide range of disciplines and professional schools. Its faculty includes approximately 2,000 professors, 88% of whom have graduated abroad; several of them have received prestigious prizes and recognition for their contribution to academic knowledge.

The Faculty of Medicine started its academic activities in 1930. In 1997, a commission of the Association of American Medical Colleges (AAMC) of the US visited the School of Medicine and examined the structure, function, and results of the Undergraduate Medical Education Program. This commission concluded that "if the School of Medicine were in the AAMC's area of jurisdiction, without doubt it would qualify for provisional accreditation based on the standards of American Schools of Medicine".

Mission statement

The Faculty of Medicine has a mission *to form physicians of science and conscience ...so that everyone that studies here be not only scientifically and technically able, but open to the different dimensions of man, and conscious of their personal and social responsibility* (Declaration of Principles).

The observance of the principles stated in the Apostolic Constitution "Ex Corde Ecclesiae" and the Declaration of Principles and Statutes of the Pontificia Universidad Catolica de Chile, represent for everyone in the university, including the academic staff, the yardstick for measuring performance.

Reproductive medicine

Professor Enrique Oyarzun, Head of the Department of Obstetrics and Gynecology, responded to the questionnaire on fertility services and research. A more extensive discussion of the challenges for reproductive medicine in Latin America is presented in Chapter X.

1. *Contraception in our Department and in our University is officially limited to the fertility awareness based methods (natural family planning). Of course all the other methods are discussed in the office between patient and physician. If the patient decides to use an intrauterine device, for example, we refer her to another center.*
2. *Female or male sterilizations are not allowed. We do not practice the so-called "uterine isolation" or sterilization at the time of Cesarean section. Nevertheless, I know that, years ago, when the physician in charge thought at the time of a Cesarean section that it was better not to have another pregnancy, they did a hysterectomy. Although this is something that was performed in the past, I can tell you that we have not done such a thing in the last twenty years. So, what we do in these cases is just to close the uterus if it does not need a hysterectomy, and advise the patient after delivery not to get pregnant again.*
3. *In our country, abortion is not permitted under any circumstances. In this matter, I need to point out that we do not consider that it is necessary to have a law permitting abortion in the following situations:*
   a) *Ectopic pregnancy;*
   b) *Co-existence of cancer of the uterine cervix and pregnancy in the first trimester;*
   c) *Partial mole with a fetus carrying a chromosomal abnormality incompatible with life;*
   d) *Clinical infection and premature rupture of membrane under 22 weeks of pregnancy;*
   e) *Severe pre-eclampsia unresponsive to treatment under 24 weeks of pregnancy.*

In all these cases we just interrupt the pregnancy because we consider, from an ethical point of view, that it is different here than in other cases. We do not consider this an abortion, because the fetal loss is a consequence of the treatment. Yet, I know that in many countries in South America that this is not the case.

4. *IVF has never been performed in our center. In those cases where our staff members in the Reproductive Medicine Unit decide that the patient needs an IVF treatment, they usually refer the patient to other centers without receiving any money, but often staying close to the patient themselves.*
5. *Our center has proved that it is possible to run an infertility clinic when IVF is not offered, being strong in diagnosis evaluation, ovarian stimulation and intrauterine insemination.*

6. *We do not have specific guidelines about some procedures that are not performed here such as donor insemination, in vitro fertilization and related techniques.*
7. *Research in reproductive medicine, in our Department, has been devoted to intrauterine insemination, post-coital test, endometriosis, evaluation of b-hCG for diagnosis and prognosis on days +15 and +23 post ovulation, ovarian stimulation and sexual intercourse timed by ultrasound follow-up.*

9. Georgetown University, Washington DC

History

Georgetown University began with the vision of John Carroll, an American-born, European-educated Jesuit priest who returned to the United States, in 1773, with the goal of securing the future of American Catholicism through education – in particular, through the establishment of pre-eminent Catholic places of higher learning. The vision of John Carroll continues to be realized today in a distinctive educational institution – a national university rooted in the Catholic faith and Jesuit tradition, committed to spiritual inquiry, engaged in the public sphere, and invigorated by religious and cultural pluralism.

The Joseph P. and Rose F. Kennedy Institute of Ethics was established in 1971. The institute is a teaching and research center offering ethical perspectives on major policy issues. It is the largest university-based group of faculty members in the world devoted to research and teaching in biomedical ethics and other areas of applied ethics.

Georgetown University Hospital was founded in 1898 to promote health through education, research and patient care. This mission has been shaped by, and reflects, Georgetown's Catholic, Jesuit identity and heritage. With a 609-licensed bed hospital and 1100 physicians, Georgetown University Hospital's clinical services represent one of the largest healthcare delivery networks in the area.

Reproductive medicine

It was not possible at the time of the inquiry for the Department Chairman to respond to the questionnaire as significant changes in governance were underway within the institution. However, the previous Chairman, Professor Craig Winkel, provided the following information (Table 29.3).

Table 29.3. Clinical services in reproductive medicine at Georgetown University

---

Contraception
- natural methods   yes
- condom   not given, but prescribed
- pill   not given, but prescribed
- IUCD   not inserted on site, but at affiliated clinics
- emergency pill   not given, but prescribed

Sterilization
- on demand   not provided on site
- medical indication   not provided on site

Abortion
- on demand   no
- socio-economic   no
- medical indication   no
- life threatening condition no

Donor insemination
- married couple   managed by outsourced RE division
- unmarried couple   managed by outsourced RE division
- single   no
- lesbian   no

Reproductive surgery   yes

In vitro fertilization
- married couple   managed by outsourced RE division
- unmarried   managed by outsourced RE division
- single   no
- lesbian   no

RE: reproductive endocrinology

The faculty of the Georgetown University School of Medicine agrees to adhere to the Catholic Directives. At the same time, there is recognition of the special relationship that exists between the physician and the patient. For these reasons, it is generally held that the "Church" does not have a place in the consultation room or the examination room. Thus, discussions of contraceptive needs, assisted reproduction, sterilization, insemination and other related topics remain within the purview of the patient-physician relationship and are not open to regulation as far as discussion goes.

The university hospital, however, does not support the performance of female or male sterilization procedures or abortion. For many years it was held to be appropriate to perform "uterine isolation" in the event that, during cesarean section, uterine dehiscence or other abnormality was indicative of future risk. In 1999, however, the performance of uterine isolation procedures was abandoned at the direction of the higher authorities in the university and the Catholic diocese.

Today, faculty members, in the course of providing care to women, regularly discuss and prescribe contraceptives (oral, as well as other forms). The hospital pharmacy does not stock oral contraceptives, condoms, etc. on site and patients must fill prescriptions for those items at retail pharmacies. Many faculty members have privileges to practice at affiliated hospitals in the Washington DC metroplex and take their patients to those other institutions to perform tubal ligation. Most of the faculty members and many of the non-faculty physicians do not have an interest in performing abortion and thus that does not seem to be an issue.

Interestingly, one of the first prenatal genetics programs in the US was developed at Georgetown University under the direction of a Jesuit scientist. That program is still in existence. Couples at risk of genetic abnormalities in the developing fetus are provided with extensive counseling and genetic testing using all of the most sophisticated modalities available. If genetic abnormalities are detected, counseling is provided. If abortion is desired, the patients are referred for services in the DC area.

Recently, in light of the increasing financial difficulties being faced by hospitals in the US, the university hospital was "leased" for 99 years to a non-Catholic hospital corporation. The agreement was signed with the proviso that the university hospital would still continue to adhere to the Catholic Directives.

The Department of Obstetrics and Gynecology provides services in reproductive medicine through Shady Grove Fertility Associates. This group runs the largest ART program in the mid-Atlantic region. They will perform approximately 1600 IVF cycles in 2005. They maintain a full-time rented office within the department at Georgetown University. The members of this group constitute the Division of Reproductive Endocrinology. They provide the full range of infertility services, but only perform monitoring, consultation, and examination on site. When oocyte retrieval and embryo transfer are necessary, those procedures are undertaken at their facility.

Medical students at Georgetown University receive the training required by the accrediting bodies. This includes lectures on contraception, abortion, and sterilization. They also participate in oral examination scenarios that involve these topics. Residents in training receive instruction and have experience in each of these areas of education also. The issue of abortion is still one of personal interest throughout the US. Residents are not required at any institution to perform abortion. However, all institutions make such training and experience available for those who request it. At Georgetown, such training is obtained at affiliate, non-Catholic hospitals.

10. Loyola University Chicago, Michigan

History

Ranked a top national university and a "best value" for education, Loyola University Chicago is one of the largest of the 28 Jesuit universities and colleges in the United States, with three campuses in the greater Chicago area, plus the Rome Center in Italy, and nine schools and colleges.

Mission of Loyola University Chicago

"We are Chicago's Jesuit Catholic university, a diverse community seeking to find God in all things and working to expand knowledge in the service of humanity through learning, justice and faith."

Loyola University Chicago embodies the four essential characteristics of a Catholic university as described in the August 1990 apostolic exhortation of John Paul II:

* *A Christian inspiration not only of individuals but of the university community as such;*
* *A continuing reflection in the light of the Catholic faith upon the growing treasury of human knowledge, to which it seeks to contribute by its own research;*
* *Fidelity to the Christian message as it comes to us through the Church;*
* *An institutional commitment to the service of the people of God and the human family in their pilgrimage to the transcendent goal which gives meaning to life. (Ex Corde Ecclesiae n. 13.)*

Mission of the Loyola University Chicago Stritch School of Medicine

* *Every medical school has unique characteristics, a distinctive personality, goals for the future.*

* *At the Stritch School of Medicine, we are committed to graduating out-standing doctors who have an exceptionally well-rounded approach to life and medicine.*

* *As a Jesuit Catholic institution, we encourage all Loyolans to uphold certain values within that religious tradition, including compassion, service and respect for life.*

Reproductive medicine

Dr. Michael Zinaman, Director of Reproductive Endocrinology and Infertility, completed the questionnaire on the clinical practice of reproductive medicine at the Stritch School of Medicine (Table 29.4).

However, the answers did not reflect the official position of the hospital or University Authority for every item. In practice, the pill and the emergency pill are prescribed for contraception. Staff members do not perform in vitro fertilization, but provisions are present for donor insemination in case of male sterility.

There is no mention on the website of the university hospital of a comprehensive infertility clinic at the Stritch School of Medicine.

Table 29.4. Clinical services in reproductive medicine at the Stritch School of Medicine in Chicago

Contraception	
– natural methods	yes
– condom	yes
– pill	yes
– IUCD	no
– emergency pill	yes
Sterilization	
– on demand	no
– medical	yes
Abortion	
– on demand	no
– socio-economic	no
– medical	no
– life-threatening condition	no

Donor insemination
- married couple   yes
- unmarried couple   yes
- single   yes
- lesbian   yes

Reproductive surgery   yes

In vitro fertilization
- married couple   no
- unmarried   no
- single   no
- lesbian   no
- egg donation   no

---

11. Saint Louis University, St Louis, Missouri

History

Saint Louis University is a Jesuit, Catholic university ranked among the top research institutions in the nation. The university fosters the intellectual and character development of 11,500 students on campuses in St. Louis and Madrid, Spain. Founded in 1818, it is the oldest university west of the Mississippi and the second oldest Jesuit university in the United States. Through teaching, research, health care and community service, Saint Louis University is the place *where knowledge touches lives.*

Mission statement

> *The mission of the Department of Obstetrics and Gynecology of the Saint Louis University School of Medicine is to achieve excellence in:*
> • *Patient care, which encompasses the primary comprehensive health care needs of women, and full spectrum specialty services with expertise in every single aspect of obstetrics and gynecology.*
> • *Research including biological investigation, clinical research and health services research.*

Reproductive medicine

According to the hospital website, the Division of Reproductive Endocrinology and Infertility provides expert diagnosis and treatment for infertile couples including cervical, ovulatory and tubal factors. There is one faculty member for the division.

The Saint Louis University School of Nursing has a Center for Fertility Education that teaches natural family planning (NFP) methods. Professional nurses who are specialists in teaching NFP provide couples with classes monthly for three months.

Dr. Michael Thomure, Director of Reproductive Endocrinology and Infertility, provided the following information on the questionnaire (Table 29.5). IVF is not performed on the premises, but IVF patients are referred to other non-Catholic universities.

Table 29.5. Clinical services in reproductive medicine at the St Louis University School of Medicine

Contraception	
– natural methods	yes
– condom	yes
– pill	yes
– IUCD	yes
– emergency pill	yes (some doctors do)
Sterilization	
– on demand	no
– medical	no
Abortion	
– on demand	no
– socio-economic	no
– medical	no
– life-threatening condition	no
Donor insemination	
– married couple	yes
– unmarried couple	yes
– single	yes
– lesbian	yes
Reproductive surgery	yes
In vitro fertilization	
– married couple	no
– unmarried	no
– single	no
– lesbian	no
– egg donation	no

30. Clinical research

The research activity in reproductive medicine at the four Catholic universities in Europe and the three Catholic universities in the US was further investigated in detail.

The search was based on the scientific medical publications in English from these seven Catholic universities during the last 25 years. The international, but not the national or regional, medical publications can be easily retrieved from search machines such as PubMed. We searched PubMed with the name of the university in combination with the terms "natural family planning", "contraception", "infertility", "sterility" and "in vitro fertilization".

In additon, a questionnaire on the use of human gametes and embryos for research was sent to the Catholic universities with an in vitro fertilization program.

Europe

Università Catholica del Sacro Cuore (A. Gemelli hospital)

The Gemelli hospital is a well-known international center for research on tubal endoscopy and reconstructive tubo-ovarian surgery, although in vitro fertilization is not accepted, even in patients with irreparable tubal damage.

According to PubMed there were no publications on natural family planning methods and in vitro fertilization, but there were 3 publications on oral contraception and 24 on infertility (Table 30.1).

Katholieke Universiteit Leuven (K.U.Leuven)

Since the mid-1970s, the K.U.Leuven in Belgium has been an international research and training center for reproductive medicine. In addition to reproductive endocrinology the center was internationally known for training and research in reconstructive reproductive surgery.

In 1996, the hospital authority reorganized the infertility services and created the Leuven University Fertility Center (LUFC). In 2005, the center qualified for the ISO 9001: 2000 management certificate attesting to the quality of the services offered by the fertility team.

In Chapter X, Jean-Jacques Cassiman, a genetic expert, describes the medical indications for preimplantation genetic diagnosis. In the same Chapter Jan Deprest and colleagues describe how endoscopic fetal surgery has developed since the early 1990s. The K.U.Leuven is now one of the leading centers of fetal surgery.

The search of PubMed revealed no publications on natural family planning, 9 publications on oral contraception, 90 on infertility and 34 on in vitro fertilization (Table 30.1).

Université Catholique de Louvain (U.C.L.)

The Université Catholique de Louvain in Belgium has a very strong international reputation for its research and training in reproductive medicine and particularly endoscopic surgery.

In Chapter X, Jacques Donnez describes recent research in the prevention of infertility in women with cancer.

The search of PubMed revealed no papers on natural family planning, 8 papers on oral contraception, 41 on infertility and 13 papers on in vitro fertilization (Table 30.1).

Radboud Universiteit Nijmegen

The UMC St Radboud in the Netherlands has been a leading international center in the field of reproductive medicine. As described in Chapter X by Tom Eskes, the research in the past focussed on the role of homocysteine in fetal development and the prevention of neural tube defects.

The search of PubMed revealed no publication on natural family planning but 10 papers on oral contraception, 90 on infertility and 40 on in vitro fertilization (Table 30.1).

Table 30.1. Publications on selected topics of reproductive medicine at Catholic universities

	NFP	Pill	Infertility	IVF
Europe				
Sacro Cuore	0	3	24	0
K.U.Leuven	0	9	90	34
U.C.L.	0	8	41	14
St Radboud	0	10	90	40
US				
Georgetown	44	5	24	1
Saint Louis	2	0	0	0
Loyola	0	0	12	0

NFP: natural family planning
IVF: in vitro fertilization

United States

Saint Louis University

PubMed revealed two publications on natural family planning (Table 30.1).

Georgetown University

The Department of Obstetrics and Gynecology has been, for many years (and still is), very active in research in reproductive medicine.

Georgetown University has numerous publications in international scientific journals on the natural family planning methods (Table 30.1).

In Chapter X, Victoria Jennings describes a new method of natural family planning that has been coined "CycleBeads". This visual method allows the identification of the fertile period of a woman's menstrual cycle. The technique has gained worldwide acclaim and was developed under a grant from USID. In addition, a new mucus-based method entitled the "TwoDay" method is also described.

Via PubMed we traced 44 papers from Georgetown University on natural family planning, 5 papers on the pill, 25 papers on infertility and 1 paper on in vitro fertilization (Table 30.1). However, staff members have published many more papers on infertility and in vitro fertilization from the outsourced location, the Shady Grove Fertility Reproductive Science Center.

Loyola University

The search of PubMed revealed that there is an interest in the study and treatment of male infertility, but otherwise no publications on the selected topics of reproductive medicine were traced via PubMed (Table 30.1).

The three Catholic universities in the Low Countries have together published a total of 336 articles on fertility and sterility in recent years, while the three catholic universities in the USA have published a total of 88 articles. On the topic of "infertility", 221 articles were published by the three Catholic medical schools in the Low Countries, while only 36 articles were published by the three major schools of medicine in the US. On the other hand, 46 articles were published on natural family planning by two Catholic schools of medicine in the US, while none were published by the four Catholic schools of medicine in Europe, including the Gemelli Hospital in Rome. These findings will be commented on in the Epilogue.

The results of the questionnaire on research involving gametes and embryos at the Catholic universities with an in vitro fertilization program are summarized in Table 30.2.

The questionnaire on research in reproductive medicine was completed at the U.C.L. by the head of the Department and at the UMC by the head of the Infertility Center.

In 2002, the Commission for Medical Ethics at the K.U.Leuven approved the donation of spare embryos for research. The embryos would become the property of a commercial spin-off company associated with the university. The frozen spare embryos could be brought back in culture for growth and development until the blastocyst stage in order to obtain stem cells for experimental research. The couples have to wave any claim to remuneration or participation in the profits in case the company takes patents.

Table 30.2. Questionnaire on research in reproductive medicine
The question was whether or not the procedure is, or can officially be, performed. If the answer is no, the personal view is rated as 1: desirable, 2: undecided or 3: undesirable.

	K.U.Leuven	U.C.L.	St. Radboud
Research on:			
– Sperms (by masturbation)	yes	yes	yes
– Preimplantation embryo	no/3	no/3	no/2
Embryonic stem cell research			
– Induced abortion tissue	no/3	no/3	no/3
– Spare embryos	yes	yes	no/2
– Embryos created by IVF	no	no/3	no/2
– Using cloning	no	no/2	no/2

31. Polarization

The most obvious result of the survey is the polarization of reproductive medicine at the Catholic universities. The polarization affects clinical services, training and research in reproductive medicine and separates sharply the progressive Catholic universities in the Low Countries from the other Catholic universities in the world. However, the polarization tends to be less extreme at some Catholic universities, where physicians are able to make arrangements for fertility services that are not officially permitted by the Hospital Authority.

Clinical services

Natural family planning (NFP) is officially the only acceptable method of contraception at orthodox Catholic universities. Several universities have set up specific services to teach couples the methods of NFP. Georgetown University has, in collaboration with Catholic universities in Latin America, a very active research program on NFP. In contrast, the Catholic universities in the Low Countries have shown very little interest in NFP in the past.

Oral contraception, emergency contraception, condom and intrauterine contraceptive device (IUCD) are not acceptable at any of the orthodox Catholic university hospitals. However, in the context of the physician-patient relationship these methods are likely to be discussed in many places. This may be less the case for emergency contraception and IUCD, which are rightly or wrongly suspected of having an abortive mechanism of action. In contrast, all modern contraceptive methods are available at the progressive Catholic universities in the Low Countries, whenever indicated. Some physicians at these universities, however, make reservations on the use of emergency contraception and IUCD for the above-mentioned reason.

Tubal sterilization is another field of polarization between progressive and orthodox Catholic universities. However, at some orthodox Catholic universities tubal sterilization is performed under the code of "uterine isolation" or accidental irreparable damage of the tubes, if during cesarean section a uterine dehiscence or other abnormality exists that is indicative of future risk. Today, gynecologists find it unethical to perform a cesarean hysterectomy for the sole purpose of sterilization. Tubal sterilization can be performed at all three Catholic universities in the Low Countries for the purpose of definitive contraception.

Abortion is not available for socio-economic reasons at any Catholic university. However, the indication for abortion can be discussed at Catholic universities in the Low Countries when there is a major medical reason or the pregnancy is life-threatening. Each case is discussed by an ad hoc committee and in the case of positive advice the procedure can be performed at these university hospitals.

At orthodox Catholic universities abortion is not available for a woman, even if her life is at risk.

Prenatal diagnosis is offered at many Catholic university hospitals. Some Catholic universities have extensive services of counseling and genetic testing for couples at risk for genetic abnormalities in the developing fetus. If genetic abnormalities are detected, further counseling on abortion is provided at these places.

Donor insemination is accepted as a treatment of male infertility at the K.U.Leuven, but not at any other Catholic university.

In vitro fertilization (IVF) is performed at the three Catholic university hospitals in the Low Countries for married as well as unmarried couples. The other assisted reproductive technologies such as intracytoplasmatic sperm injection (ICSI), preimplantation genetic diagnosis (PGD) and cryopreservation of embryos are also available at these places.

Georgetown University in the US has a special arrangement by outsourcing in vitro fertilization. This means that the fertility physician is allowed to perform counseling, ovarian stimulation and monitoring on the premises of the university hospital, but egg aspiration, in vitro fertilization, embryo transfer and other assisted reproductive techniques are performed at premises outside the university hospital. Obviously, the University Authority carries no responsibility for the "unorthodox" practices of the academic staff outside the university premises. The arrangement means that Georgetown University has an experienced staff in reproductive medicine, that junior doctors can receive full theoretical and practical training, and that research on IVF and allied techniques is performed on the premises outside the Catholic university. In an attempt to continue fertility services physicians at some orthodox Catholic universities make arrangements with outside IVF centers and refer their patients to these centers for the IVF procedures.

In vitro fertilizaton with sperm and egg donation is officially accepted at the K.U.Leuven, but not at any other Catholic university.

In vitro fertilization in lesbian couples, single women or with a gestational carrier is not acceptable at any Catholic University.

Clearly, reproductive medicine is restricted at all Catholic university hospitals. The Hospital Authorities at orthodox Catholic universities follow strictly the restrictions as imposed by the Church Directives. A survey of the effect of the Church Directives on the physician-patient relationship in reproductive medicine has, to the best of our knowledge, not been performed. The pressure to follow the Church Directives in the office and the operating room appears to have increased during recent years in the US. Control of the office practice by pressure groups, which may use undercover informants, has been reported in the US. In 1999, Georgetown University abandoned the practice of tubal sterilization at the time of cesarean section in patients at risk during a future pregnancy.

Reproductive medicine at the Catholic universities in the Low Countries is also restricted, but significantly less than at orthodox Catholic universities. These universities are clearly not following the "Instruction on Respect for Human Life in its Origin and the Dignity of Procreation" issued by the Sacred Congregation for the Doctrine of the Faith in February, 1987. In March/April 1987, the Catholic universities of Lille (France), Leuven (Belgium), Louvain-la-Neuve (Belgium) and Nijmegen (The Netherlands) issued a declaration stating that the efforts to integrate the new technologies of assisted reproduction into a human context should not be discontinued. Both Catholic universities of Leuven and Nijmegen regretted that they were not included in the wide consultation, which was claimed to have resulted in the 'Instruction' issued by the Sacred Congregation.

Clinical research

Research in reproductive medicine, as in any other branch of medicine, is essential for improving our understanding of human reproductive ecology and the quality of reproduction. Research can improve the modalities of new therapies and address the medical as well as the ethical issues, which may arise during the development of a new technology. Major medical and ethical issues in reproductive medicine, particularly in association with in vitro fertilization, are addressed by appropriate clinical and basic research.

Unfortunately, research in reproductive medicine cannot be performed if there is no clinical service. The search of PubMed confirms that the Catholic universities which strictly follow the Church directives, no longer have comprehensive infertility clinics and are no longer active in fertility research. In contrast, the program of training and research in fertility and infertility is flourishing at the three Catholic universities in the Low Countries. Moreover, as shown in Chapter X, the orientation of research at these universities is fully in line with the spirit of prevention of diseases and improving the quality of reproduction.

It can be concluded that the Church directives are increasingly incompatible with the practice and teaching of modern reproductive medicine. The conflict has resulted in a disorganization and even disintegration of infertility services at most orthodox Catholic university hospitals. The demand for infertility treatment at these universities has largely dwindled away, unless provisions were made for outsourcing the services or referring patients to external IVF centers. On the other hand, the progressive Catholic universities have integrated modern contraceptive methods and assisted reproductive technologies in a Christian and human context. These universities are providing a range of clinical services in fertility and infertility, which are apparently well accepted by the patients in their respective countries.

CHAPTER X
RESEARCH ORIENTATION

This chapter presents a scientific anthology which is typical for the research orientation in reproductive medicine at Catholic universities. Victoria Jennings' contribution illustrates the outstanding research efforts in natural family planning. Enrique Ayurzon analyzes the challenges for a high-quality reproductive medicine at Catholic universities in Latin America. Tom Eskes stresses how prevention of birth defects is an excellent topic to work on within a Catholic framework that addresses both medico-biological and ethical issues. Other challenging innovative research subjects at Catholic universities are fertility preservation for female patients with malignancies as described by Jacques Donnez and collaborators, and reconstructive endoscopic fetal surgery, described by Jan Deprest and co-investigators. Jean-Jacques Cassiman, an expert in human genetics, outlines the possibilities and drawbacks of preimplantation genetic diagnosis in clinical practice.

32. Natural family planning: the TwoDay Method™

Victoria Jennings, Georgetown University, US

Introduction

Natural family planning (NFP) is based on the observation of the fertile and infertile periods of the menstrual cycle. Couples using natural methods are aware when sexual intercourse can result in pregnancy and can time intercourse according to their pregnancy intentions. While many couples who use NFP do so to achieve pregnancy, the focus of this chapter is on pregnancy avoidance.

Successful use of natural methods depends on three factors:

1. The accuracy of the method in identifying the woman's fertile period;

2. The ability of the couple to use the method correctly to determine the woman's fertile time; and
3. Their ability and willingness to avoid sexual intercourse when the woman is fertile.

Well-established NFP methods, such as the Billings Ovulation Method and the Symptothermal Method (and their variants), have been carefully studied to determine their effectiveness in helping couples avoid pregnancy. These methods are very effective when used correctly.[1,2] Furthermore, their use poses no potential harm to either the woman[3] or – should pregnancy occur – to the developing fetus.[4] These methods are now offered through NFP programs (primarily related to the Catholic Church) in countries around the world. The Billings Ovulation Method involves daily observation of cervical mucus to assess its characteristics, recording of mucus observations on a chart, and application of method rules to determine when the woman is fertile. The Symptothermal Method involves similar mucus observations, plus daily recording of basal body temperature and application of method rules.

Despite their efficacy and safety, the acceptance and use of these methods is limited. Estimates from surveys conducted in many countries indicate that an extremely small percentage of women are using NFP methods, and these numbers have fallen in most countries during the last decade.[5] Researchers have suggested that some of the reasons for this limited use include the time and effort required to train NFP teachers (some training programs involve a few weeks of training, others involve several months); the time required to teach a couple to use NFP (ranging from several hours to several days over a period of three to six months); and the complexity of using the methods.

Nonetheless, there is a large unmet need for family planning that can be partially addressed by the availability of natural methods that are easy to teach, easy to learn and easy to use. Surveys show that, worldwide, over 30 million women report that they are using "periodic abstinence" to prevent pregnancy.[6] The great majority of them, however, do not know when they are most likely to get pregnant, making their efforts to avoid pregnancy often unsuccessful. Additionally, millions of women who do not want to get pregnant are not using any method of family planning. Others are using a method inconsistently, switching methods frequently, or discontinuing a method after just a few months.

With this in mind, researchers at Georgetown University's Institute for Reproductive Health, with support from the United States Agency for International Development, have developed two new natural methods, the Standard Days Method™ (SDM) and the Two-Day Method™ (TDM). These methods are discussed in terms of their development, efficacy, service delivery issues, and current status.

The Standard Days Method

The SDM, like other natural methods, is based on the physiology of the menstrual cycle and the functional life span of the sperm and the ovum. It is appropriate for women whose menstrual cycles are usually between 26 and 32 days long (approximately 80% of cycles are within this range)[7]. Couples using the SDM are advised that the woman should be considered fertile on days 8 through 19 of her cycle.

Method development:

In developing the SDM, researchers considered two probabilities: the probability of pregnancy *vis-à-vis* ovulation, and the probability of the timing of ovulation *vis-a-vis* mid-point of the cycle.

With regard to the first probability, hormonal and ultrasound studies have shown that a woman is fertile up to a total of six days each cycle – five days before ovulation plus the 24 hours after ovulation.[8] There is approximately a 4% probability of pregnancy from intercourse five days before ovulation. This increases to 15% four days before ovulation. The highest probability of pregnancy – between 25% and 28% – is on the two days before ovulation. During the 24 hours after ovulation, there is an 8–10% probability. Fertility then decreases, with a 0% probability of pregnancy by the day after ovulation. (See Figure 32.1.)

These probabilities are due to the limited viable life span of the sperms after ejaculation (not more than five days) and to the very limited viable life span of the egg following ovulation (less than 24 hours). Together these result in an actual fertile window of no more than six days during the woman's cycle. On all the other days, the woman cannot become pregnant.

In determining when ovulation occurs, and thus when during the cycle the six-day fertile window occurs, researchers again considered probability. Data has shown that in the great majority of cycles, ovulation occurs very close to the middle of the cycle, particularly in cycles between 26 and 32 days long.[9] In approximately 30% of cycles,

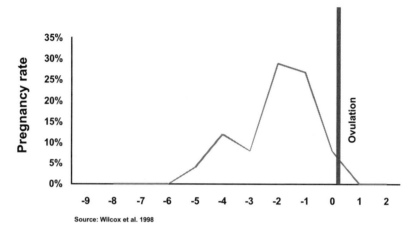

Figure 32.1. Probability of pregnancy from intercourse on days relative to ovulation.

ovulation occurs at the mid point (for example, on or very close to day 14 in a 28-day cycle, or day 15 in a 30-day cycle). In approximately 60% of cycles, ovulation occurs within one day before or after mid cycle. And in approximately 78% of cycles, ovulation occurs within two days before or after the midpoint. By four days before or after the midpoint, 95% of ovulations have occurred. (See Figure 32.2.)

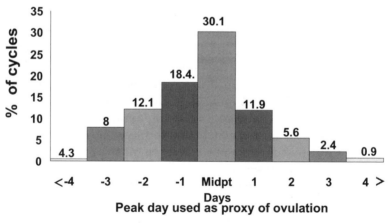

Figure 32.2. Probability of ovulation relative to midpoint of the cycle.

Researchers then created a computer model based on the combination of these two probabilities – the probability of pregnancy on different cycle days related to ovulation, and the probability of the timing of ovulation. They applied this model to a large data set provided by the World Health Organization, which included more than 7500 menstrual cycles, and found that, for women with menstrual cycles between 26 and 32 days long, pregnancy is likely only on days 8 through 19 of the cycle. On all other days, pregnancy is very unlikely. Therefore, it was suggested that to use the Standard Days Method to prevent pregnancy, couples avoid intercourse from day 8 through day 19 of each cycle. On all the other cycle days, they can have intercourse without concern of pregnancy.[10]

Efficacy study

Once the SDM was established "in theory", an efficacy study was conducted, with the approval of the Georgetown University Institutional Review Board. Some 478 women participated in the multi-center prospective study. Study participants were between 18 and 39 years old, had at least one child, had not used a hormonal method of family planning for at least two months, were determined to have regular menstrual cycles (defined as most cycles between 26 and 32 days long, as assessed by a screening protocol), stated that they and their husbands were willing and able to avoid intercourse for 12 consecutive days each cycle and wanted to delay pregnancy for at least one year, and were assessed at very low risk for sexually transmitted diseases and contraindications of pregnancy.

Before the study began, service providers in programs including Ministry of Health clinics and non-governmental organizations were trained to offer the SDM. Most providers had little or no previous experience with natural methods. The method was provided in a single counseling session during which the woman (or the woman and her husband) was taught how to use the SDM. To assist them with method use, they were given CycleBeads™, a visual tool that represents the menstrual cycle (see below for details).

Women were entered into the study as soon as they began to use the SDM, that is, immediately after being instructed in the method. (Unlike most studies of NFP efficacy, there was no "learning phase" in which the early cycles of use and the pregnancies that occur during them were excluded from the study.) Correct use of the method (i.e., accurately identifying cycle day, determining whether it is fertile or infertile, and avoiding intercourse on fertile days) was quite high: the method was used correctly in approximately 95% of cycles. About one-half of the participants completed 13 cycles of method use. The most common reason for leaving the study was having two cycles outside the 26 to 32 day range during the study period (28%). Fewer than 4% left the study because they or their husband did not like the method. There were a total of only 43 pregnancies in 4035 cycles of use. Most pregnancies occurred during cycles in which couples had unprotected intercourse during days 8 through 19. Significantly, more than 40% of pregnancies occurred during the first three cycles of method use.

Single-decrement multi-censoring life table analysis was used to determine pregnancy rates. The first-year pregnancy rate was 4.5 (95%: CI 2.33–7.11) with correct use, and 12 (CI 8.47–15.33) taking into account all cycles and all pregnancies.[11]

Service delivery issues:

Several additional studies of the SDM have been conducted, and research continues in several areas. Perhaps the most important finding is that CycleBeads is an essential component of teaching and use of the method.

CycleBeads is a color-coded string of beads that help a woman keep track of her cycle days, know which days she can get pregnant (days 8 through 19), and monitor her cycle lengths to be sure they are between 26 and 32 days long. To use CycleBeads, she moves a rubber ring over one bead every day to visibly track where she is in her menstrual cycle. The colors of the beads indicate whether she is on a fertile or infertile day. Couples are counseled to avoid intercourse when the rubber ring is on a white bead, representing a fertile day. Figure 32.3 describes how to use CycleBeads.

Following are additional findings that are helpful to programs that want to include the SDM in their services.

• It is very important for a woman to be screened, preferably by a provider, before she begins using the SDM to assess whether her cycles are likely to be between 26 and 32 days long. While it is not necessary for her to know her exact cycle length, her response to two questions ("Do your periods usually come about a month apart?" and "Do your periods usually come when you expect them?") are sufficient for this assessment.[12]

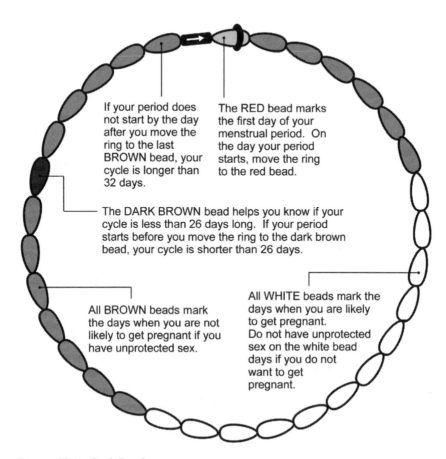

Figure 32.3. CycleBeads.

- On-going monitoring of cycle length also is important, as some women have less regular cycles than they initially believe. The SDM is not as effective for women with cycles outside the 26 to 32 day range.[13]
- The SDM can be offered in a wide range of programs, from NFP programs to those involved in community development, as well as in both the public and private sectors.
- The SDM can be used successfully by both low-literacy and high-literacy women.
- Most people who choose the SDM do so because it is natural and has no side-effects. Religion appears to be a very minor factor in choosing this method.

- Different kinds of providers – from skilled clinicians to community health workers – can teach the SDM successfully. While experienced clinical providers may need less than three hours of training, lower-level providers may require up to two days. However, their ability to counsel women and couples in the method is quite similar.
- Including the SDM in programs can expand significantly the numbers and kinds of clients reached. Programs that offer only NFP are finding that their clientele increases dramatically when they include the SDM, as are those that offer a wider range of methods. In general, the number of users of other methods (including other natural methods) does not decrease, suggesting that the SDM is "additive" rather than absorbing clients who otherwise would have used another method.

Current status

The SDM is now being used in more than 25 countries around the world. Ministries of health, non-governmental organizations, international private voluntary organizations, and community development groups are including it in their policies, norms, and services. The method is included in international guidance documents such as the World Health Organization's *Medical Eligibility Criteria for Contraceptive Use*[14], USID's *Global Health Technical Briefs*[15], and *Contraceptive Technology, 18th edition*[16]. Materials for training and service provision, including an on-line training for providers, are available from the Institute for Reproductive Health website www.irh.org.

The Twoday Method

To address the major limitation of the SDM, which is that only women with regular cycles between 26 and 32 days can use the method, Georgetown University researchers developed the TDM. The TDM, like a number of other natural methods, uses cervical mucus as the indicator of fertility. However, it does not involve analyzing the characteristics of the mucus (e.g., amount, color, consistency, slipperiness, stretchability, viscosity, etc.), and the method rules are quite simple. To use the TDM, women monitor themselves each day to determine whether or not they have any mucus that day. Then they ask themselves two questions:

- Did I notice any secretions today?
- Did I notice any secretions yesterday?

If any secretions were noticed on either of the two days she will potentially be fertile. If no secretions were noticed on either day (two consecutive days with no secretions), the probability of becoming pregnant that day is very low. (See Figure 32.4.)

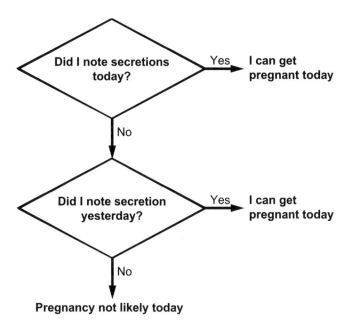

Figure 32.4. The TwoDay algorithm.

Couples using the TDM should avoid intercourse on days when the woman is potentially fertile.

Method development

As with the SDM, researchers first determined the theoretical efficacy of the TDM by applying the algorithm described above to existing data sets – the 7500 cycles from the World Health Organization and a data set from an Ovulation Method center in Vicenza, Italy. Results of this analysis indicated that the theoretical efficacy of the TDM was at least as high as that of the SDM.[17] Subsequent analyses confirmed these results.[18]

Efficacy study

A prospective, multicenter study, approved by the Georgetown University Institutional Review Board, was undertaken to test the efficacy of the TDM. A total of 450 women were admitted to the study. The sample included women aged 18–39 years who had at least one previous child, had not used hormonal contraception during the previous two months, and were assessed to be at low risk of sexually transmitted diseases and pregnancy complications. In addition, all participants and their husbands wanted to delay pregnancy for at least one year and were were willing to avoid intercourse on days the TDM identified as fertile.

The method was offered through existing health care programs. The Institute for Reproductive Health trained five to ten health service providers, most without previous experience with natural methods, in each site to offer the TDM. These providers screened potential participants for study eligibility, counseled participants in the TDM, and collected the data. Participants were first taught how to monitor their cervical mucus. Providers explained that the mucus might look or feel different on different days of the cycle and that amounts of mucus vary, but that the woman should consider herself fertile if she noticed mucus of any type, regardless of characteristics or amount. Women were interviewed every cycle to assess their use of the method and their pregnancy status. However, instruction in the TDM was limited to the initial counseling session and a single follow-up session.

Of the 450 participants who entered the study (women entered the study following their initial counseling session), more than half completed 13 cycles of method use. Using single-decrement multi-censoring life table analysis, the first-year pregnancy rate with correct use of the method was 3.5 (95% CI 1.44–5.52). When all cycles and pregnancies were included in the analysis, the pregnancy rate was 13.7 (95% CI 9.93–17.34).

Incorrect method use was reported in approximately 4% of the 3920 cycles in this study. Incorrect use had three potential sources: inaccurate observations of the presence or absence of cervical mucus, inaccurate application of the two-question algorithm, and having intercourse on a day identified as fertile by the method rules. A total of 47 pregnancies were reported, mostly during the first three cycles of use and in cycles in which couples had intercourse on days identified by the method as fertile.[19]

Service delivery issues

The efficacy study provided important information that can help programs and providers offer the TDM to clients. In addition to the finding that women were able to identify the presence or absence of cervical mucus and to apply the two-question algorithm, several additional findings are of interest:

- Users of the TDM gained confidence in their ability to use the method over time;
- Counseling women to note the presence or absence of cervical mucus "after noon" and "just before going to bed at night" is adequate for identifying fertile days;
- Community-based and clinic-based providers are equally competent in counseling women in the method.

Current status

Following the efficacy study, materials for providers and users of the TDM were developed and tested, based on recommendations from efficacy study participants. These materials are available from the Institute for Reproductive Health website, www.irh.org.

Additional studies are underway to compare the effect of starting to use the TDM at various times in the menstrual cycle on accurate understanding and correct use.

The TDM is included in the World Health Organization's *Medical Eligibility for Contraceptive Use*.[20]

Conclusion

Both the SDM and the TDM are effective and easy-to-use natural methods that appeal to a wide range of couples. These methods can address a critical unmet need for family planning in both developed and developing countries, and offer additional choices to women and men who want to use a natural method of family planning.

References

1. Guida M, et al, An overview on the effectiveness of natural family planning, *Gynecol. Endocrino*, (1997) 203–219.

2. Trussell J, Grummer-Strawn L. Contraceptive failure of the ovulation method of periodic abstinence. *Family Planning Perspectives*, (1990) 65–75.

3. Improving Access to Quality Care in Family Planning: Medical Eligibility Criteria for Contraceptive Use, 2nd edition. World Health Organization, 2003.

4. Simpson JL, Gray R, Perez A, Mena P, Queenan JT, Barbato M, Pardo F, Kambic R, Jennings V. Fertilization involving aging gametes is not associated with major birth defects and Downs Syndrome. *Lancet* 2001 (359);9318:1670-1671.

5. Demographic and Health Surveys, Reproductive Health Surveys, various. 1994–2004.

6. Population Reference Bureau. World Population Data Sheet, 2004.

7. Arevalo M, Jennings V, Sinai I. A fixed formula to define the fertile window of the menstrual cycle as the basis of a simple method of natural family planning. *Contraception*, 2000; 60:357–360.

8. Wilcox A, Weinberg C, Baird D. Post-ovulatory aging of the human oocyte and embryo failure. *Human Reproduction*, 1998; 13:394–397.

9. Arevalo et al, 2000, op cit.

10. Arevalo et al, 2000, op cit.

11. Arevalo M, Jennings V, Sinai I. Efficacy of a new method of family planning: the Standard Days Method. *Contraception*. 2002;65:333–338.

12. Sinai I, Jennings V, Arevalo M. The importance of screening and monitoring: the Standard Days Method and cycle regularity. *Contraception*, 2004;69:201–206.

13. Sinai I, et al, 2004, op cit.

14. World Health Organization, op cit.

15. Global Health Technical Briefs, *The Standard Days Method: a Simple, Effective natural Method*, US Agency for International Development, 2004.

16. Hatcher R, et al. *Contraceptive Technology*, 18th edition, 2004. Ardent Media, New York, NY.

17. Sinai I, Jennings V, Arevalo M. The TwoDay Algorithm: a new algorithm to identify the fertile time of the menstrual cycle. *Contraception*. 1999;60:65–70.

18. Dunson D, Sinai I, Colombo B. The relationship between cervical secretions and the daily probabilities of pregnancy: effectiveness of the TwoDay Algorithm. *Human Reproduction*, 2001;16:2278–82.

19. Arevalo M, Jennings V, Nikula M, Sinai I. Efficacy of the new Two-Day Method of family planning. *Fertility and Sterility*. 2004; 82(4): 885–892.

20. World Health Organization, op cit.

33. Challenges for reproductive medicine at Catholic universities in Latin America

Enrique Oyarzún
Pontificia Universidad Catolica de Chile, Chile

Introduction

The scope of this article is to discuss some of the challenges facing physicians working in a Catholic university medical school in the field of reproductive medicine. However, before so doing it is important to provide the reader with some information about reproductive health in South America.

Maternal health in the Americas

Latin America is the region of the world with the greatest health inequalities between countries and between people living in individual countries. In the year 2000, the GDP (Gross Domestic Product) of Latin American countries varied between $ 3210 in Ecuador and $ 12,791 in Argentina. Chile, with its GDP at $ 9623, is placed among the wealthier countries spending 7.2% of GDP on health, while other countries spend from 2.4% to 10.9% (Uruguay). In 1997, in Chile there were 110 physicians per 100,000 inhabitants (with 10 gynecologists per 100,000 inhabitants).

Within Latin America, Chile has the highest level of antenatal care and of institutional deliveries attended by skilled personnel. Furthermore, our rates of maternal and infant mortality, and percentages of premature deliveries and low-weight newborn babies, are the lowest in Latin America.

Chile was the only country in America that, in the year 2000, reached the objective, established in 1990, of reducing maternal mortality by 50%. In the year 2003, Chile reached the lowest maternal mortality in its history, practically equal to that of the United States and the objective set by WHO for the year 2015 seems at hand.

Chilean bio-demographic success has been reached thanks to several factors: wide provision of antenatal care with different levels of attention depending on specific needs, skilled attendance at delivery, complementary maternal feeding, use of corticosteroids and of surfactants in premature labor, a significant drop in fertility rates and, since 2000, pregestational folic acid supplementation. It has to be emphasized that such successes have been achieved with a contraceptive coverage only marginally over 50% (56% in 1998), a rate lower than that of other countries in the region and without the legalization of abortion.

In the Sexual Rights Workshop, which was held in Santa Cruz de la Sierra (Bolivia), in October 2002, obstetrics and gynecology societies throughout the continent promised to work to reach the following objectives for their women: a satisfactory sexual life, free of violence and of the risk of acquiring diseases or undesired pregnancy; the right to safe pregnancy and delivery; and the right to freely decide about controlling their fertility, including through pregnancy interruption if the legislation of the country permitted it. There is no doubt that the sexual and reproductive rights of women constitute an inseparable part of the set of human rights confirmed by different international statements, as well as in the constitutions of most countries of the world.

In many countries, including Chile, there are major obstacles that still prevent the full inclusion of women in the social, political, and economic life. In the same way that certain groups have advocated abortion legalization, as a matter of justice, we also need to advocate free and safe motherhood, improving the social and working environment in which women live, recognizing that mankind owes its own survival to the ability of women to go through pregnancy and delivery without risks.

Today, gender equity also demands full support for those women who, with heroic love for their baby, go ahead with a pregnancy even when it is the consequence of violence and rape. And, certainly, we must also take care of all those that, undergoing pressures of a different nature, terminate their pregnancy. Today, public opinion seems set to eliminate the idea that voluntary abortion is intrinsicly evil, although, in most cases it is the woman's own conscience that prevents her from forgetting that the life of her own child has been taken away, because her predisposition to welcome life is encoded in her mind from time immemorial. These women should not be punished, on the contrary, they must be cared for as Pope John Paul II indicated in the Encyclical letter Evangelium Vitae:

I want to have a special reflection for you, women who have resorted to an abortion. The Church knows the situations that probably influenced your decision, and knows that in many cases yours has been a painful and even dramatic decision. Probably the wound has not even healed in your heart. It is the truth that what happened was and continues to be deeply unjust. Nevertheless, do not let yourselves be taken by discouragement and do not abandon hope.... the Father of all mercy waits for you to offer His pardon and His peace to you in the sacrament of Reconciliation. You will realize that nothing is lost and you will also be able to ask pardon to your son who now lives in God.

Reproductive health in Chile

The situation in Chile is very different from that prevailing in the rest of the Latin American continent. Table 33.1 summarizes general data of this country.

Table 33.1

Population	15.116.435	(2002)
GDP	9.623 USD	(2000)
Population growth rate	1.17	
General mortality rate	5.5 per 1000 inhab.	(2000)
Life expectancy at birth	Male 72.4 years Female 79.2 years	(2000)
Birth mortality rate	8,9 per 1000 live births	(2002)
Inhabitants per doctor	841	(2004)
Public health system budget 2004	2500 millions USD	
Schools of medicine	21	
Literacy rate	96%	

Recent surveys show that 80% of the population in Latin America claims to be Catholic, and as such, bioethical and legal considerations are influenced by Catholic principles. There are issues in which our university has made clear statements, although other Catholic universities look more flexible.

In 1968, Chile became the first country in Latin America to have a national program for fertility regulation, and oral contraceptives and intrauterine devices are delivered free of charge to most of the population served by the national health system.

Science is growing at a pace never heard of before. The amount of knowledge we have gained since we graduated is staggering and mind-boggling. There is also an increasing dependence of medicine on technology. For each new discovery, many new questions arise. In recent years, burning issues in the world have been the human genome, cloning, surrogate motherhood, gene manipulation, emergency contraception, life support in the terminally ill and euthanasia.

Challenges

Our challenge is to meet modern societies' increasing requests for specialized and high-quality health services, as it is to be expected from an industrialized, technologically developed, globalized and medium-high economical level country.

Today's society requires physicians who are able to learn and think scientifically, apply their knowledge, and serve society as a whole. Nevertheless, physicians must be moulded not only intellectually, but also morally, ethically and attitudinally. Our school needs to stimulate and promote charity, solidarity, human dignity, freedom and social justice.

A Catholic medical school should reflect its catholicity in its mission, academic programs, and clinical practices. Attributes that should distinguish a Catholic medical school are an emphasis on medical ethics in academic and research programs; service to the poor and underserved; high standards of professionalism and recognition of the importance of spirituality in medicine.

Catholicity presents challenges that other medical schools may not face. These can occur around medical practices and research methods that, although accepted by many in our society and allowed under the law, are contrary to Catholic teaching. Examples are abortion, contraception, embryonic stem cell research, and physician-assisted suicide. A Catholic medical school must maintain a clear position on these matters. But we believe in academic freedom and respect each individual's choice and freedom of conscience. Nevertheless, those who think differently are expected to respect the principles of the university and when they speak or act on behalf of a Catholic university, they have to respect the identity of the institution.

For those of us who believe in the transcendent nature of human beings and in the absolute value of our unique dignity, a medical action is acceptable only when it is performed to preserve human life or to improve the quality of human life. By contrast, any medical procedure that does not respect human life and the dignity endowed to every single person is considered unacceptable.

We face a major challenge in believing that the above mentioned principles are part of an absolute truth; we need to find an answer to the options offered today by medical progress which are the elements that serve or contradict those principles. Our final goal is to protect human life. But, we need to achieve a balance between being faithful to the doctrine and social and medical demands.

Final thoughts

There are many topics that have not been addressed in this chapter, but we do believe that in the future many of them will need to be discussed in our various countries.

There are, today, dilemmas regarding contraception, including sterilization and emergency contraception; confidentiality regarding reproductive issues in adolescent care; infertility treatment and questions ranging from the way sperm samples are obtained to the limitation in the use of some of the available techniques; prenatal diagnosis; induced abortion, including "therapeutic abortion"; genetic counseling; HIV/AIDS prevention; managed care, and the problems that arise when the public system and /or health care institutions have a "joint venture" with a Catholic hospital; how to deal with the international guidelines and rules that the Government has signed and agreed to respect (Beijing); respect for conscious objection, and others.

After all, a Catholic institution needs to be coherent between what it teaches and what it does. This is an especially sensitive issue when you have teaching facilities within the same private practice.

The Catholic university should contribute to the society within which it is situated with a service of evangelization of culture that is based on a conception of man and in an integral teaching of the person. Integral teaching means growth as a person in every way. A university can train excellent physicians, but a Catholic university has, additionally, to prepare them to face up to ethical and moral problems that arise during the practice of their profession. Research and treatments in a Catholic university must always be undertaken with a concern for the moral and ethical implications of the methods and the new scientific discoveries. Moreover, priorities need to be determined, and for most of the countries of the Latin American region, modern reproductive technologies, for example, are not the most important action to be implemented.

Further reading

Paulo VI, Enciclica Humanae Vitae (1968)
Ciudad del Vaticano, congregación para la Doctrina y la Fe, Instrucción
　　sobre el respeto a la Vida Humana Naciente y la Dignidad de la Pro-
　　creación (1987)
Ryder R E "Natural family planning": effective birth control supported
　　by the Catholic Church. *BMJ* 1993; 307:723–6
Juan Pablo II, Evangelium Vitae (1995)

34. Periconceptual prevention of neural tube defects

Tom Eskes, K.U.Nijmegen, NL

Summary
Birth defects can be prevented by the use of folic acid or folic acid
enriched food in the periconceptional period.

Introduction

Sex and reproduction at Catholic universities encompasses a combination of medicine, biology and medical ethics.

I was Professor and Chairman of the Department of Obstetrics and
Gynecology at the Catholic University in Nijmegen (St. Radboud
Hospital) from 1972 to 1998. During this period prenatal diagnostics
was introduced to protect the rights of the unborn child. The only
problem was that there was frequently no therapy for a negative
diagnosis, and both the couple and the doctor would be forced to
decide on a "medical" abortion.

It was at this point that our thought became focussed on primary
prevention because prevention is better than cure.

Primary prevention of birth defects

Birth defects can occur in virtually all organs and limbs of the human
body. They arise in the first months of pregnancy. We decided to
focus our attention on defects of the brain and spinal cord. The reason for this was the publication of a paper by Professor Smithells and
collaborators of Leeds (UK) entitled: "Possible prevention of neural-
tube defects by periconceptional vitamin supplementation". This

study was challenging because the use of multivitamins reduced neural tube defects ten times!

Spina bifida: a birth defect with serious handicaps

Spina bifida belongs to the so called neural tube defects. Our brain and spine are already formed from the 15th day after conception onwards as an open tube. This tube has to close in the next few days, so very early in pregnancy (day 15-28 after conception / one to two weeks after the expected menstruation). If closure does not happen at the top of this tube a great part of the brain and skull will be absent. This defect is called anencephaly and is lethal; if the tube does not close at the tail side the lower part of the spine will remain open with damaged nerves for the bladder, the rectum and the legs (spina bifida). This results clinically in incontinence for urine and faeces. The legs are paralyzed.

Spina bifida: birth rates and prenatal diagnosis

The birth prevalence rate of neural tube defects varies between countries, socioeconomic and ethnic groups. The numbers range from 1:2500 in Finland, 1:700 in the Netherlands, 1:300 in Mexico and 1:80 in Wales. These figures are estimates because the number of legal abortions for neural tube defects is not known.

Worldwide around 400,000 children are born per year with an open neural tube defect (NTD).

Spina bifida can be diagnosed during pregnancy by the determination of alpha-fetoprotein and acetylcholinesterase in amniotic fluid and by ultrasound.

Spina bifida: the cause

For years it was suspected that some metabolic condition in the mother caused spina bifida because this defect occurred especially in poor areas. The first indication for this was when Stein et al (1975) found, during the examination of patients, that those who were conceived during the Dutch hungerwinter 1944–1945 had a significant number of open spines.

Spina bifida can also result from anti-epileptics or anticancer medication.

A rather constant number of cases are due to chromosomal anomalies (trisomy 13 or 18, triploidy translocations), or specific syndromes (Meckel and Robert syndrome).

An important phonecall: multivitamins

I phoned Professor Smithells and made an appointment for a personal interview. In Leeds I met a devoted pediatrician who was willing to discuss all details of his study. When I asked him why he did not perform a placebo-randomized study his answer was that the medical ethical commissions of the co-operating hospitals did not allow him to do so. The reasoning was that Smithells had found some vitamin deficiencies in women with NTD offspring and the committee suggested that. "When you diagnose such a deficiency you should supplement that".

Smithells was not sure which vitamin was important. His hypothesis was folic acid.

Folic acid

In 1930, folic acid was first recognized as a factor present in the yeast preparation Marmite, which was able to cure a megaloblastic anemia occurring among Hindu women in India during pregnancy. The term 'folic acid' comes from the Latin word folium which means leaves. The substance was successfully synthesized in 1941.

In food the vitamin is present as a molecular structure with more than one side chain and is called folate. Folate has to be reduced to one side chain to be biologically active. Furthermore, folate is heat labile. That means that around 70% of it will be destroyed by cooking.

The synthetic form is a molecule with only one side chain and is therefore immediately active.

Most studies in the literature are done with folic acid in tablet form.

Folic acid and folate belong to the important B-vitamins and is categorized as vitamin B11. This vitamin is present in all sorts of "mediterranean food" but also in meat, milk products, bread, potatoes and liver.

Folates and folic acid can be determined in blood.

Folates are present in all body tissues. Folate is stored to the greatest extent in erythrocytes, the liver, pancreas, kidneys and brain.

History of spina bifida

Neural tube defects were already known to the Egyptians and drew continuous attention in every century because of the enigma of birth defects.

One of the first detailed pictures of spina bifida was made in 1641 by Nicholas Tulp, a disciple of Rembrandt. Tulp was the Mayor of Amsterdam, but also a doctor and painter.

Studies in Nijmegen (NL)

• *Vitamin profiles do not identify women likely to have offspring with NTD.* After a site visit to Leeds and a grant from the Dutch Prevention Foundation it was possible to raise a new and modern vitamin laboratory.

The first results of our study in the Netherlands were disappointing: Dutch women with NTD offspring did not differ in their blood vitamin profiles from controls. Also folate levels did not differ.

This was in sharp contrast with Smithells' findings.

• *Derangement of homocysteine metabolism is the possible basis for neural tube defects.*

Through further study in the literature and working with dedicated researchers I learned that folic acid was the motor of the so called methionine-homocysteine metabolism. Methionine and homocysteine are small sulphur-containing amino-acids that have to furnish (in co-operation with vitamin B12) methylgroups (CH3) for the building and expression of DNA in each cell (Figure 34.1). The necessary methylgroups are delivered by methylfolate with the co-operation of Vitamin B12.

With this knowledge in mind it was logical to have another look at the mothers of NTD offspring focussing on homocysteine / methionine metabolism.

Steegers-Theunissen et al were the first from our research group to report on a possible derangement of folate dependent homocysteine metabolism in women who had NTD offspring. When women had a high level of homocysteine their risk of having a child with NTD was almost seven times higher.

This finding was extended and confirmed in the international literature and served as a catalyst for further studies.

Homocysteine with its rather "naked" sulfur atom turned out to be the causal agent, damaging the embryonic process as well as the inner lining of blood vessels.

Methionine had the methylgroup at the sulfur atom making it less aggressive and more friendly by donating methylgroups that were received from folic acid and vitamin B12.

It was also found that some women with NTD offspring had genetic mutations. Fortunately folic acid administration could overcome this genetic failure (in contrast to many other genetic diseases).

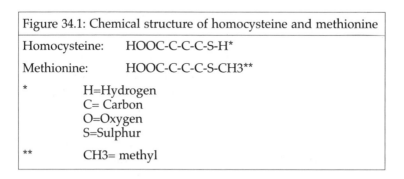

Figure 34.1: Chemical structure of homocysteine and methionine
Homocysteine: HOOC-C-C-C-S-H*
Methionine: HOOC-C-C-C-S-CH3**
*   H=Hydrogen C= Carbon O=Oxygen S=Sulphur
**   CH3= methyl

• *Folate and homocysteine metabolism (fig 34.2)*

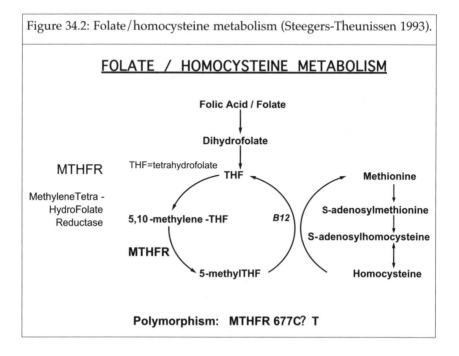

Figure 34.2: Folate/homocysteine metabolism (Steegers-Theunissen 1993).

FOLATE / HOMOCYSTEINE METABOLISM

Folic Acid / Folate

Dihydrofolate

MTHFR

THF=tetrahydrofolate

THF

MethyleneTetra - HydroFolate Reductase

5,10 -methylene -THF   B12

MTHFR

5-methylTHF

Methionine

S-adenosylmethionine

S-adenosylhomocysteine

Homocysteine

Polymorphism: MTHFR 677C? T

Folic acid or folate are transformed via dihydrofolate into THF (tetrahydrofolate). From THF 5,10 methylene- THF is formed.

The next step is crucial: The enzyme MTHFR (methylenetetrahydrofolate) facilitates the formation of 5-methylTHF. The appearance of a methylgroup is essential here because this methylgroup will be used to form DNA.

With the help of Vit B12 5-methylTHF goes either into THF or into methionine. Between methionine and homocysteine there is an exchange of methylgroups.

The human body avoids accumulation of homocysteine because of its toxicity. When folate stores are adequate homocysteine levels will be low and vice versa.

• *Genetic mutations in women with NTD offspring*
Each step of this biochemical circuit is speeded up by enzymes. Enzymes are proteins and are formed through DNA codes. When these codes are wrong (mutations) the proteins of enzymes will be less active or not active at all.

So far most studies report on mutations of MTHFR: in this gene on chromosome 1 there is a substitution of amino acids (the building blocks of proteins) at nucleotide 677. The Nijmegen research group was the first to report on MTHFR mutation in women with NTD offspring (van der Put et al).

In summary we can state that the crucial finding of the Nijmegen research group was that homocysteine was a critical parameter of folate status, when lowered it was a risk factor for NTD and could be accompanied by genetic mutations.

Folic acid supplements are clearly capable of lowering plasma homocysteine concentrations.

• *Homocysteine is toxic for the embryo*
In the laboratories of toxicology at the medical faculty in Nijmegen it was possible to study the whole rat-embryo in vitro. In the incubator it could be demonstrated that homocysteine had embryotoxic properties. Serine, vitamin B12 and 5 –methyl THF could ameliorate this toxicity. This confirmed what was suspected clinically.

This research can also be considered a tribute to Vincent du Vigneaud, late Professor of Biochemistry at the Cornell University Medical College and Nobel Prize Winner for the discovery and synthesis of the uterostimulant oxytocin. He was one of those pioneers who recognized the importance of sulfur-containing amino-acids, their transsulfuration and transmethylation.

Folic acid alone or embedded in a multivitamin prevents neural tube defects

At the same time that we discovered the importance of homocysteine for the pathogenesis of NTD, the Medical Research Council in the United Kingdom published the results of a large multicenter, double-blind, randomized trial in which the possible effect of multivitamins and folic acid on the recurrence rate of neural tube defects was studied.

This study fulfilled all the criteria for an excellent randomized investigation. Daily supplementation with folic acid (4 mg/d), folic acid (4 mg/d) with other vitamins, other vitamins without folic acid and placebo, led to a 72% reduction of the recurrence rate in the folic acid groups.

The rationale for the choice of such a high dose of folic acid was to avoid the risk of an ineffective low dose and the impossibility of repeating such a long-lasting and costly study. The trial was closed prematurely because of the conclusions reached before the calculations were completed.

From an ethical point of view it is remarkable to note that Smithells did not get permission from the ethical committees to perform a placebo-randomized trial and that the Medical Research Council did not even mention ethical consultation. Nevertheless we can be quite satisfied with the results.

The Hungarian randomized trial by Czeizel and Dudás also provided evidence that the occurrence of neural tube defects could be prevented. Subjects took a daily multivitamin containing 800 mcg folic acid per day. The control group used a placebo containing trace elements. It could not be disclosed if the significant result was due to folic acid alone or to folic acid embedded within the multivitamin preparation.

One has to realize that the MRC and the Hungarian study were performed in a rather high-prevalence area for neural tube defects.

Other birth defects: congenital heart disease, orofacial clefts, miscarriage and Down's Syndrome

Birth defects, recognized as anatomical abnormalities at birth, affect 8 million children per year worldwide. Neural tube defects and congenital heart anomalies rank high.

The neural crest plays a major role in the development, outgrowth and fusion of the neural walls and the migrating neural crest cells are also involved in the heart "anlage" and in the closure of the midline. Therefore studies were initiated to unravel the possible role of homocysteine in the etiology of congenital heart defects and cheilo-palato schisis.

Further studies demonstrated that mothers had offspring with birth defects of the cardiovascular system (Kapusta et al), orofacial clefts (Wong et al) and early miscarriage (Nelen et al). In all these studies maternal hyperhomocysteinemia and genetic mutations were present.

Homocysteine levels could be lowered by the use of folates or folic acid and when genetic mutations were present. This was one of the first examples of nature-nurture interaction.

Hobbs CA et al reported on abnormal folate metabolism in Down's Syndrome (Am J Hum Genet 2000; 67: 623).

Folate supplementation around conception therefore has the potential to reduce the frequency of Down's Syndrome. This finding strengthens the recommendation to use folic acid around conception in addition to the prevention of neural tube defects.

This is a major step forward towards the causes and prevention of this syndrome.

Food fortification with folic acid and the use of folic acid in tablets around conception

Since 1998 the US government has enriched cereal grains with folic acid.. In 2004, it could be stated that folic acid prevented around 50% of NTD's.

The Health Council of the Netherlands did not advise the government to enrich food. Some of the members were afraid of side-effects (these however, do not occur when folic acid is given in a dose lower than 1 mg).

The percentage of women that used folic acid in the proper way was 4.8% in 1995. This percentage rose to 35.6 in 2000.

In our own area we could reach a percentage of 52%.

The contribution of the Prevention Foundation and Corporate Development International (CDI) to the Nijmegen research group

Research is impossible without well-trained and enthusiastic personnel. At a university it is always possible to find such personnel but it is not so easy to find sponsors.

CDI contributed to our research with a yearly contribution of around € 15000,00. This enabled us to start a project and to apply for larger grants allowing a researcher to work on the project for four years.

The Prevention Foundation and the Foundation Catholic University sponsored us up to a total of around three million Euro.

The research group produced 125 papers in high-ranking scientific journals and 14 PhD's.

Summary

Primary prevention of birth defects is an excellent topic to work on at a Catholic university. It combines medico-biological with ethical issues.

A multidisciplinary research group was installed in Nijmegen (NL) in the eighties*. This group demonstrated that mothers with neural tube defect (spina bifida) offspring had a derangement of folate- and homocysteine metabolism and genetic mutations.

This was also found for congenital heart disease, schisis, recurrent early miscarriage and Down's Syndrome.

Homocysteine is a very sensitive indicator for the folate status. Homocysteine plasma values have to be low because they are embryotoxic. High values can be lowered by folic acid and also food folate in women with genetic mutations, demonstrating nature-nurture interaction.

Folate (vitamin B11) is the motor of methionine-homocysteine metabolism and provides methyl (CH3) groups for DNA synthesis.

Placebo-randomized studies in the UK and Hungary demonstrated, in 1991 and 1992, that folic acid could prevent up to 72% of the recurrence and occurrence of neural tube defects.

There is now observational evidence that folic acid can prevent a wide range of birth defects other than those of the neural tube. This approach avoids legal abortion.

The next step will be to convince women that it is necessary to take folic acid before and around conception or to enrich food.

* The research described in this article was sponsored by the Prevention Foundation, the Foundation Catholic University and Corporate Development International. It contributed to the primary prevention of birth defects by describing the underlining basis of folic acid administration. The research output on birth defects, homocysteine and folate/folic acid from 1983 till 2004 by the Nijmegen research group was 13 PhD theses and more than 125 scientific articles.

References

PhD theses from the Catholic University Nijmegen (NL):

Mooij PNM (1992) Vitamins, Folate and Reproduction: a study in
    humans and animals
Steegers-Theunissen RPM (1993) Homocysteine, Vitamins and Neural-
    Tube Defects
Van Aerts LAFG (1995) Embryotoxic studies on cyclophosphamide and
    homocysteine
Wouters MGAJ (1996) Recurrent miscarriage and hyperhomocystinemia
Blatter B (1997) Spina bifida and parental occupation
Den Heijer M (1997) Hyperhomocysteinemia and venous thrombosis
Kluijtmans L (1998) Molecular genetic analysis in hyperhomocysteinemia
Van der Put N (1999) Homocysteine, Folate and Neural Tube Defects
Brouwer I (1999) Folic acid, folate and homocysteine: human interven-
    tion studies
Hol FA (1999) Genetic factors in human neural tube defects
Nelen WDLM (2000) Risk factors for recurrent early pregnancy loss:
    Hyperhomocystinemia, thrombophilia and impaired toxification
Van Rooij IALM (2003) Etiology of orofacial clefts
Groenen P (2004) Nutritional and environmental factors in human spina
    bifida: an emphasis on myo-inositol
Klootwijk ED Inositol and zinc related neural tube defects. Genetic, mor-
    phological and supplementation studies in mouse. Human genetic
    studies

Further reading

Carmel R, Jacobson DW (2001) Homocysteine in health and disease
    Cambridge University Press
Massaro EJ, Rogers JM (2002) Folate and human development. Humana
    Press Totowa, New Jersey

35. Transplantation of cryopreserved ovarian tissue

Jacques Donnez, U.C.L., Belgium

Introduction

The life-saving treatment endured by cancer survivors provokes, in
many cases, early menopause and subsequent infertility. In clinical
situations where there is often a pressing need to start chemotherapy,

ovarian tissue cryopreservation looks to be a promising option to restore fertility.

It has been estimated that, by 2010, one in 250 people in the adult population will actually be childhood cancer survivors .[1] The treatment of childhood malignancy is becoming increasingly effective. Aggressive chemotherapy and radiotherapy, as well as bone marrow transplantation, can cure more than 90% of girls and young women affected by such malignancies. However, the ovaries are very sensitive to cytotoxic treatment, especially to alkylating agents and ionizing radiation, generally resulting in the loss of both endocrine and reproductive function.[2] Moreover, it is known that uterine irradiation at a young age reduces adult uterine volume.[3]

There are several potential options available to preserve fertility in patients facing premature ovarian failure, including immature and mature oocyte cryopreservation, embryo cryopreservation and cryopreservation of ovarian tissue.[4,5] For those patients who require immediate chemotherapy, cryopreservation of ovarian tissue is a possible alternative.[4,6,7]

History of experimental and clinical studies

To date, ovarian tissue has been successfully cryopreserved and transplanted in mice and rodents, as well as large animals like sheep and marmoset monkeys.[8-10] The first successful fertilization and pregnancy following egg collection from freshly transplanted ovarian tissue in a primate was recently described.[11] The grafted tissue functioned without any surgical connection to major blood vessels. Experimental studies have indicated that the decrease in the number of primordial follicles in grafted tissue is due to hypoxia and the delay before reimplanted cortical tissue becomes revascularized. The loss of primordial follicles in cryopreserved ovarian tissue after transplantation is estimated to be 50–65% in some experimental studies.[7,8,12] In one experimental study, in which ovarian cortex was grafted onto the uterine horn and under the skin, the loss was found to be more than 90%.[13]

Oktay et al have reported laparoscopic transplantation of frozen-thawed ovarian tissue to the pelvic side wall[14], to the forearm[15] and, more recently, beneath the skin of the abdomen. A four-cell embryo was obtained from 20 oocytes retrieved from tissue transplanted to the latter site, but no pregnancy occurred after transfer.[16] Radford et al reported on a patient with a history of Hodgkin's disease treated by chemotherapy, in whom ovarian tissue had been biopsied and cryopreserved four years after chemotherapy and later reimplanted.[17] In this case, histological section of ovarian cortical tissue revealed only a few primordial follicles because of the previous chemotherapy. After reimplantation, the patient had only one menstrual period.

We have described a live birth after orthotopic autotransplantation of cryopreserved ovarian tissue. Our findings suggest that cryopreservation of ovarian tissue should be offered to all young women diagnosed with cancer.[18]

Freeze-thawing

Freezing of ovarian tissue was carried out according to the protocol described by Gosden et al.[6] The biopsies were immediately transferred to the laboratory in Leibovitz L-15 medium supplemented with Glutamax (GIBCO, Paisley, Scotland). There, the remaining stromal tissue was gently removed.

Four biopsies of the cortex were then cut into 70 small cubes of 2x2mm. One strip of 12x4mm was left whole. Fragments (cubes and a strip) of ovarian tissue were suspended in the cryoprotective medium. All the fragments were placed into precooled 2ml cryogenic vials (Simport, Quebec, Canada) filled with Leibovitz medium supplemented with 4mg/ml of human serum albumin (Red Cross, Brussels, Belgium) and 1.5mM DMSO (Sigma, St. Louis, MO). The cryotubes were cooled in a programmable freezer (Kryo 10, Series III; Planer, Sunbury-on-Thames, United Kingdom) using the following program: (1) cooled from 0°C to -8°C at -2°C/min; (2) seeded manually by touching the cryotubes with forceps prechilled in liquid nitrogen; (3) cooled to -40°C at -0.3°C/min; (4) cooled to -150°C at -30°C/min, and (5) transferred to liquid nitrogen (-196°C) immediately for storage.

Reimplantation of ovarian cortical tissue

In 1997, a 25-year-old woman presented with clinical stage IV Hodgkin's lymphoma. Ovarian tissue cryopreservation was carried out before chemotherapy. Written informed consent was obtained. Using laparoscopy, five biopsies, about 1.2–1.5cm long and 5mm wide, were taken from the left ovary. Removing the whole ovary was not an option, as one can never completely exclude recovery of ovarian function after chemotherapy. Indeed, premature ovarian failure after chemotherapy is age-, drug- and dose-dependent and does not occur in 100% of cases.

After laparoscopy, the patient received MOPP/ABV hybrid chemotherapy (mechlorethamine, vincristine, procarbazine, prednisone, adriamycin, bleomycin, vinblastine) from August 1997 to February 1998, followed by radiotherapy (38 grays). She became amenorrheic shortly after the initiation of chemotherapy. The levels of follicle-stimulating hormone (FSH), luteinizing hormone (LH) and estradiol (E_2) following chemo- and radiotherapy were, respectively, 91.1 mIU/ml, 85 mIU/ml and 17 pg/ml, confirming castration. This ovarian failure profile was confirmed three months later. Hormone replacement therapy (HRT) was started in June 1998 and then stopped in January 2001, as the patient wished to become pregnant. A thorough evaluation by oncologists demonstrated that she was disease-free.

After cessation of HRT, FSH, LH and 17 β-estradiol levels returned to levels consistent with ovarian failure. From January 2001 to December 2002, the patient experienced only one ovulatory cycle proved by a progesterone level of 10 ng/ml and the presence of a corpus luteum on the left ovary, diagnosed by vaginal echography. The decision to reimplant was therefore taken.

A first laparoscopy was carried out seven days before reimplantation in order to create a peritoneal window by means of a large incision just beneath the right ovarian hilus, followed by coagulation of the edges of the window. The goal was to induce angiogenesis and neovascularization in this area. Both ovaries looked atrophic. Nevertheless, a small corpus luteum was visible on the left ovary. A decrease in LH and FSH was observed and the concentrations then returned to castrated levels.

A second laparoscopy was carried out seven days after the creation of the peritoneal window. A biopsy of 4–5mm in size was taken from each of the atrophic ovaries in order to check for the presence or absence of primordial follicles. The thawed ovarian cortical tissue was then placed in sterile medium and immediately transferred to the operating theatre. The large strip and 35 small cubes of frozen-thawed ovarian tissue were pushed into the furrow created by the peritoneal window very close to the ovarian vessels and fimbria on the right side. No suture was used. An extensive neovascular network was clearly visible in this space.

A third laparoscopy was carried out four and a half months after reimplantation to evaluate the survival of the graft. A follicle was visible at the site of reimplantation. Biopsy was performed. The grafted tissue was biopsied and histology and fluorescent probe staining revealed the presence of viable primordial follicles and a follicular structure with inhibin A-marked cells. Follicles at an early growth stage require more than 85 days to reach the antral stage.[19] Primordial follicles obviously require even more. The appearance of the first follicle in the grafted tissue five months after reimplantation is totally consistent with the expected time course. This time interval observed in our study between implantation of cortical tissue and the first estradiol peak (five months) is also consistent with data obtained from sheep and human beings[8,17].

From five to nine months after reimplantation, ultrasonography revealed the development of a follicle followed by corpus luteum formation with each cycle, at the site of reimplantation. This corresponded to an estradiol level of more than 100 pg/ml and a progesterone level ranging from 12 to 37 ng/ml. The LH and FSH levels were significantly ($p<0.05$) lower than those observed before reimplantation. This led to the restoration of consecutive menstrual bleeding each month.

At nine and a half months, FSH levels increased to 78.7 mIU/ml and returned to normal values seven days later. Three weeks later, a follicle of 2.6cm in size had developed on the right side, clearly outside the right ovary. Both native ovaries were well visualized and found to be obviously atrophic. Eighteen days after ovulation, calculated by basal body temperature, the hCG level was 2853 mIU/ml.

We cannot explain this sudden and temporary surge in FSH. It is possible that it was associated with a decline in inhibin secretion, as suggested in the sheep model[20,21] or with slower follicular growth from a poor follicular reserve in the graft. Indeed, due to the loss of primordial follicles in the transplant, the follicular density per mm³ was low but, in any case, the total amount of cortical tissue transplanted is relatively unimportant. After transplantation, the patient would have been considered a poor responder as, of the 500 to 1000 primordial follicles that would have been transplanted, more than 50% would have been lost due to hypoxia.[12]

Is it risky?

Unfortunately, in the majority of cases, aggressive chemotherapy and radiotherapy lead to ovarian failure. The restoration of ovarian function after chemotherapy or radiotherapy has two main goals: to improve quality of life and restore reproductive function. For those patients who require immediate chemotherapy, ovarian tissue cryopreservation, performed before cancer treatment is begun, may be a means of preserving fertility without delaying the initiation of chemotherapy. However, one major concern surrounding the use of ovarian cortical strips for orthotopic autotransplantation is the potential risk that the frozen-thawed ovarian cortex might harbour malignant cells which could induce a recurrence of the disease after reimplantation. Shaw et al reported that ovarian grafts from AKR mice could transfer lymphoma to recipient animals.[22] Nevertheless, more recent studies have suggested that ovarian tissue transplantation in Hodgkin's disease is safe.[23,24,25]

In our study, histological evaluation of ovarian cortex before and after reimplantation demonstrated the absence of disease. But confirming the absence of malignant cells by light microscopy may not be sufficient, especially in other types of cancer (especially hematogenous or systemic neoplasms).[9] Screening methods to detect minimal residual disease must be developed to eliminate the risk of cancer cell transmission with reimplantation.[5]

Lines of evidence

1. The patient experienced, in total, three ovulatory cycles over a period of more than two years. All of them originated from the left native ovary. This was proved by laparoscopy and/or echography.

2. The native right ovary never demonstrated any ovarian activity at all (no follicles, no corpus luteum).

3. Even if we cannot absolutely exclude the presence of isolated follicles in the atrophic ovary, their density must be very low since serial sections of four large biopsies of atrophic ovaries failed to detect any.

4. Laparoscopy proved, by direct visualization, the development of a follicle from the grafted tissue five months after reimplantation.

5. Biopsy proved, by histologic examination, not only the survival of primordial follicles in the grafted tissue, but also the maturation of a follicle (granula-cells marked by inhibin-A). This is the first time that survival of primordial follicles has been histologically proved after cryopreserved ovarian tissue transplantation.

6. After follicular development was proved by laparoscopy and histology, the patient experienced regular menstrual bleeding. The progesterone level was systematically more than 10ng/ml in the mid-luteal phase, calculated on the basis of BBT.

During each ovulatory cycle (from five to nine months), vaginal echography demonstrated a corpus luteum on the grafted tissue outside the right atrophic ovary, which had demonstrated no ovarian activity for almost three years.

7. Finally, vaginal echography revealed the presence of a preovulatory follicle at the reimplantation site during the cycle leading to the pregnancy, but no follicles were seen on either of the native ovaries. This argument is a crucial one.

Conclusion

This is the first report of the birth of a healthy infant, obtained after orthotopic autotransplantation of cryopreserved ovarian tissue. It opens new perspectives for young cancer patients facing premature ovarian failure. Ovarian tissue cryopreservation should be an option offered to all young women diagnosed with cancer, in conjunction with other existing options for fertility preservation such as immature oocyte retrieval, in vitro maturation of oocytes, oocyte vitrification or embryo cryopreservation.

Even if more and more papers are now describing the restoration of ovarian function after orthotopic transplantation of fresh and frozen ovarian tissue and the first live birth has recently been reported, we should still bear in mind that many questions remain unanswered. In our department, research is presently under way on freezing an entire ovary. A recent paper by our group described not only the technique, but also the high rate of survival of primordial follicles after freeze-thawing an entire ovary.[26,27] This could lead to the transplantation of an intact ovary, with microvascular anastomosis carried out to restore immediate vascularization and minimize post-transplantation ischemia responsible for the reduction in follicular density. A major limitation of intact organ transplantation, which needs to be investigated, is the problem of storage of an intact ovary with its vascular tissue. Other issues, like the question of the optimum number of grafts and hence oocytes, how long the graft will last and the optimum technique and site, must be addressed.

References

1. Blatt J. Pregnancy outcome in long-term survivors of childhood cancer. Med Pediatr Oncol 1999; 33:29–33.
2. Donnez J, Godin PA, Qu J, Nisolle M. Gonadal cryopreservation in the young patient with gynecological malignancy. Current Op Obstet Gynecol 2000; 12:1–9.
3. Larsen EC, Schmiegelow K, Rechnitzer C et al. Radiotherapy at a young age reduces uterine volume of childhood cancer survivors. Acta Obstet Gynecol Scand 2004; 83:96–102.
4. Donnez J, Bassil S. Indications for cryopreservation of ovarian tissue. Hum Reprod 1998; 4:248–259.
5. Rao GD, Chian RC, Son WS et al. Fertility preservation in women undergoing cancer treatment. Lancet 2004; 363:1829–1830.
6. Gosden RG, Baird DT, Wade JC, Webb R. Restoration of fertility to oophorectomised sheep by ovarian autografts stored at –196°C. Hum Reprod 1994; 9:597–603.
7. Meirow D, Fasouliotis SJ, Nugent D et al. Laparoscopic technique for obtaining ovarian cortical biopsy specimens for fertility conservation in patients with cancer. Fertil Steril 1999; 71:948–91.
8. Baird DT, Webb R, Campbell BK et al. Long-term ovarian function in sheep after ovariectomy and transplantation of autografts stored at –196°C. Endocrinology 1999; 140:462–41.
9. Meirow D, Yehuda DB, Prus D et al. Ovarian tissue banking in patients with Hodgkin's disease: is it safe? Fertil Steril 1998; 69:996–998
10. Candy CJ, Wood MJ, Whittingham DG. Restoration of a normal reproductive lifespan after grafting of cryopreserved mouse ovaries. Hum Reprod 2000; 15:1300–1304.
11. Lee DM, Yeoman RR, Battaglia DE et al. Live birth after ovarian tissue transplant. Nature 2004; 428:137–138.
12. Nisolle M, Casanas-Roux F, Qu J et al. Histologic and ultrastructural evaluation of fresh and frozen-thawed human ovarian xenografts in nude mice. Fertil Steril 2000; 74:122–9.
13. Aubard Y, Piver P, Cognié Y et al. Orthotopic and heterotopic autografts of frozen-thawed ovarian cortex in sheep. Hum Reprod 1999; 14:2149–2154.
14. Oktay K, Karlikaya G. Ovarian function after transplantation of frozen, banked autologous ovarian tissue. N Engl J Med 2000; 342:1919.
15. Oktay K, Economos K, Kan M et al. Endocrine function and oocyte retrieval after autologous transplantation of ovarian cortical strips to the forearm. Jama 2001; 286:1490–1493.
16. Oktay K, Buyuk E, Veeck L et al. Embryo development after heterotopic transplantation of cryopreserved ovarian tissue. Lancet 2004; 363:837–840.

17. Radford JA, Lieberman BA, Brison D et al. Orthotopic reimplantation of cryopreserved ovarian cortical strips after high-dose chemotherapy for Hodgkin's lymphoma. Lancet 2001; 357:1172–1175.
18. Donnez J, Dolmans MM, Demylle D et al. Livebirth after orthotopic transplantation of cryopreserved ovarian tissue. Lancet 2004; 364:1405–1410.
19. Gougeon A. Dynamics of follicular growth in the human: a model from preliminary results. Hum Reprod 1986;1:81–87.
20. Callejo J, Salvador C, Miralles A et al. Long-term ovarian function evaluation after autografting by implantation with fresh and frozen-thawed human ovarian tissue. J Clin Endocrinol Metab 2001; 86:4489–4494.
21. Campbell BK, Telfer EE, Webb R, Baird DT. Ovarian autografts in sheep as a model for studying folliculogenesis. Mol Cell Endocrinol 2000; 163:131–139.
22. Shaw JM, Bowles J, Koopman P et al. Fresh and cryopreserved ovarian tissue samples from donors with lymphoma transmit the cancer to graft recipients. Hum Reprod 1996; 11:1668–1673.
23. Kim SS, Radford JA, Harris M et al. Ovarian tissue harvested from lymphoma patients to preserve fertility may be safe for autotransplantation. Hum Reprod 2001; 16:2056–2060.
24. Kim SS, Battaglia DE, Soules MR. The future of human ovarian cryopreservation and transplantation: fertility and beyond. Fertil Steril 2001; 75:1049–1056.
25. Kim SS. Ovarian tissue banking for cancer patients. To do or not to do? Hum Reprod 2003; 18:1759–1761.
26. Martinez-Madrid B, Dolmans MM, Van Langendonckt A, Defrère S, Donnez J. Freeze-thawing intact human ovary with its vascular pedicle with a passive cooling device. Fertil Steril 2004; 82: 1390–1394.
27. Martinez-Madrid B, Dolmans MM, Van Langendonckt A, Defrère S, Van Eyck AS, Donnez J. Ficoll density gradient method for recovery of isolated human ovarian primordial follicles. Fertil Steril 2004; 82:1648–1653.

36. Preimplantation genetic diagnosis

Jean-Jacques Cassiman, K.U.Leuven, Belgium

Introduction

In 1990, following some preliminary experiments in animals, the first publication on the clinical use of preimplantation genetic diagnosis

(PGD) appeared in the highly rated scientific journal *Nature,* opening the way for the development of new applications. In the following 15 years, more than 1000 children were born after undergoing the procedure successfully in the pre-embryo stage. This was 6 years before the cloning of animals and humans could even be reasonably considered. The study of human embryonic stem cells removed from fertilized eggs in excess of the clinical need for infertility treatment was not yet an issue of discussion.

The original methodology has been substantially improved and as a result the number of errors or unclear results have decreased substantially. While the follow up, over many years, of the children who underwent the procedure has not detected any significant increase in developmental problems, one should keep in mind that most of these children were the result of an in vitro fertilization procedure, mainly ICSI, which might carry a small risk of some developmental problems.

Sampling methods

Depending on the indications for PGD, different methods have been used to biopsy the egg or the fertilized egg immediately, or a few days after, fertilization.

Polar body biopsy

Two approaches have been followed. In the first of these, the first polar body of an unfertilized egg is removed, after mechanical or laser incision of the zona pellucida of the egg. This body carries the 23 still doubled chromosomes, which have been extruded from the egg as a result of the first meiotic division. If the woman is a carrier of a genetic defect, this defect will be either retained on the chromosomes of the egg or will be extruded with those of the first polar body. The absence of the defect in the polar body is therefore a good indication that the egg will carry the defect.

The second approach will remove the second polar body of the fertilized egg. At this time the egg, as a result of fertilization, will have extruded a second polar body containing 23 half chromosomes, which are identical to the 23 half chromosomes which will participate in the fusion with the genetic material of the male. If the defect is present in the second polar body, this means that the egg carries the defect also.

The Chicago group that pioneered this approach and appears to be able to determine the correct genetic make up in 98% of the biopsies.

The advantage of studying the second polar body is that one will obtain a result, which is a correct reflexion of the genetic constitution of the maternal contribution to the fertilized egg.

The disadvantage of this approach is, of course, that only the maternal genetic contribution is examined. This is therefore a useful approach when a dominant disease gene e.g. for Huntington's disease, carried by the mother, is the indication for the PGD. For recessive diseases, for which both parents have to contribute a disease gene to the fertilized egg for the child to be affected, the polar body approach would lead to the elimination of all affected, as well as of all carriers of the disease gene. This is statistically 75% of all fertilized eggs and would mean an important wastage of potentially good candidate eggs.

Blastomere biopsy

The most frequently used method to biopsy the fertilized egg is the removal of one or two blastomeres, three days after fertilization and in vitro culture, when the fertilized egg has completed its third division and is composed of eight blastomeres. At this time the genome of the embryo is fully represented in all cells.

The method most used will dissolve the zona pellucida locally with acid or will drill a hole in it with a laser beam. One or two blastomeres are then gently aspirated in a biopsy pipette introduced through this hole and can then be examined for defects. Whether the removal of more than one cell from the pre-embryo affects the implantation and development of the embryo is not clear.

Very few attempts to biopsy the blastocyst at day five have been attempted. While more cells can be taken at that stage there are a number of reasons why this method is not very popular: the fertilized egg will only rarely develop to the blastocyst stage in vitro; the diagnosis has to be rushed since the blastocyst has to be returned to the uterus before day six in order to have a reasonable chance to implant.

Analysis of the genome

Polymerase clain reaction (PCR)

The region of the genome under investigation can be selectively amplified using the polymerase chain reaction. Specific oligonucleotide primers complementary to the beginning and the end of the

DNA fragment containing the defect will allow one in a few hours to make millions of copies of this fragment. This is done in an appropriate buffer containing nucleotides, a DNA polymerase and divalent cations. Once the amplified fragment has been obtained, different methods to visualize the defect can then be applied, including sequencing of the whole fragment.

The two main problems encountered in this phase of the investigation are contamination with exogenous DNA and allele-drop out (ADO). Contamination with PCR products hanging around in the lab or with the DNA of the investigator can only be avoided using rigorous cleaning methods on all equipment used in the procedure and strict operating procedures. Before ICSI was used to fertilize the egg, contamination of the sample with spermatozoa still sticking to the zona pellucida occurred regularly. Cumulus cells also need to be carefully removed.

Allele-drop out is the non-amplification of one of the two alleles of the DNA fragment, thereby giving the false impression that the pre-embryo is either heterozygote for the defect or not affected.

Both contamination and ADO can be identified by amplifying other DNA fragments, which carry polymorphisms that characterize the two genes under investigation and/or to amplify other DNA fragments with polymorphisms characteristic of the two parents of the embryo such as the HLA genes. This is usually done in a single multiplex amplification step. This will require that the four alleles present in the parents are carefully studied before PGD is initiated. Real-time PCR, which allows semi-quantitative analysis of the PCR product, will also detect ADO.

Fluorescent in situ hybridization (FISH)

Fluorescent in situ hybridization allows one to hybridize a fluorescent DNA probe composed of DNA specific for one chromosome to a non-dividing blastomere nucleus and thus to visualize the number of a particular chromosome present in the cell. The more fluorochromes that can be used simultaneously, the more chromosomes that can be examined. At present, kits containing probes for the chromosomes X, Y, 13, 16, 18, 21 and 22 are available, which can be hybridized simultaneously on the same cell. This allows one to detect the sex of the embryo, trisomies and monosomies for specific chromosomes, which are very common (up to 80%) in the embryos that do not implant or abort spontaneously.

If a more detailed analysis of the chromosomes is required, such as in the case of chromosome translocation carriers, the cells will have to be in mitosis to visualize each chromosome more accurately. FISH can then be used to visualize the translocation. This method, while very useful on chromosome preparations from peripheral blood, requires good quality chromosome spreads, which is rarely obtained for a single blastomere and prolongs the period needed to obtain a result.

Whole genome amplification

In recent years, methods have become available to amplify the whole genome of a single cell by PCR. This approach has the advantage that the analysis of chromosome abnormalities and of gene defects can be done on the same cell, which is not the case for FISH and PCR, which are mutually exclusive. The method needs further optimization for single cell DNA, however, to determine its exact failure and success rate on single cells.

Comparative genome hybridization (CGH)

Comparative genome hybridization measures the number of copies of DNA fragments present on one chromosme. For this purpose, the DNA of the chromosome is amplified and labeled with a fluorochrome, e.g. green. It is then mixed with the amplified DNA of a control sample labeled with a different fluorochrome, e.g. red. The mixture is then hybridized to a chromosome spread and the color ratio measured. A yellow signal indicates an equal proportion of control and sample DNA hybridizing; a green signal indicates an excess of the sample DNA (trisomy), while a red signal indicates a lack of sufficient sample DNA (monosomy). The advantage of this method over FISH is that regional differences within one chromosome can be identified. The disadvantage is the time required to do the whole analysis (about three days).

CGH can also be used to examine thousands of DNA fragments from the genome simultaneously. The whole genome is then amplified and labeled, mixed with control amplified DNA and hybridized to a micro array containing thousands of DNA fragments from the genome. In this case, a yellow dot will indicate equal proportions of control and sample DNA, while red will be equal to a deletion and green to a duplication or trisomy of a specific DNA fragment. While this method is still experimental in its application to PGD, there is no doubt that it could become a method of choice once the time to prepare the samples and to obtain the results has been reasonably reduced and when the exact limits of the method will be known for single cell samples.

Indications and results

In principle, all genetic defects for which the responsible gene has been identified, and for which the parents have been shown to be carriers, can be detected by PGD. In practice, the number of diseases for which PGD has been applied is still limited. The main reason for this is that for each gene defect, the PCR will have to be carefully developed and validated before PGD can be offered. Indeed, unless all disease-causing mutations are the same in a particular gene, a couple-specific PCR will have to be developed before PGD can be attempted.

This is, of course, not the case for the detection of chromosome aneuploidies (trisomies, monosomies), which is indeed applied more frequently than the detection of gene defects.

A second reason that the number of diseases that are being analyzed by PGD is limited is that the number of centers in Europe that can offer such testing is still limited and in some countries, such as Germany, is even not available because of legal limitations.

A last reason why PGD is still to be considered an experimental method is that only couples who have opted for PGD will, providing all other conditions are fulfilled, be offered PGD. Indeed, one should not forget that PGD can only be done in the context of an in vitro fertilization procedure, which is not necessarily the first choice of couples to become pregnant, unless they have been traumatized by a previous prenatal diagnosis experience or by a traumatic experience with a family member suffering from the disease.

Monogenic diseases

Cystic fibrosis, an autosomal recessive disease resulting in a life-threatening dysfunction of the airways and the digestive tract, is by far the disease for which most PGDs have been performed in the world. The fact that this disease is frequent (about 1 in 3600 births in the Caucasian population) and that the gene was identified more than 15 years ago, is probably the main reason for this.

ß thalassemia, and sickle cell anemia, spinal muscular atrophy, Huntington's chorea, achondroplasia, myotonic dystrophy, and retinoblastoma are other examples of reasonably frequent indications.

In total, about 30 different monogenic diseases have already been studied, be it sometimes singly or in a limited number of cases. The molecular expertise of the center, which offers PGD will, of course, be an important determining factor in the choice of the disease that can be considered for these tests.

A special group is formed by the X-linked diseases, such as Duchenne muscular dystrophy, Lesh Nyhan syndrome (HGPRT deficiency), fragile X mental retardation and hemophilia. Initial attempts at PGD used only sexing as a tool to identify potentially affected males. In view of the risk that carrier females could be symptomatic, such as in fragile X syndrome and in view of the fact that these genes have now been identified, a direct analysis of the gene has become the method of choice for these diseases. Nevertheless, sexing can be a last resort solution, when the gene test is too complex or the couple is already at an age where waiting for the development of a new test would decrease their chances on a successful pregnancy substantially.

Chromosomal defects

Aneuploidy in the fertilized egg increases exponentially with the age of the mother (from about 1% under the age of 34 to over 50% at the age of 45). Moreover, more than 70% of abnormally developing embryos carry chromosome anomalies and up to 60% of the early clinical pregnancies carry a major chromosome anomaly. These findings have stimulated the use of FISH, as described above, in PGD to detect trisomies, monosomies and polyploidies in the embryo (PGD-AS or PGD aneuploidy screening), even in the absence of any other indication for PGD. Chromosome analysis has therefore become a way to control the quality and viability of the embryo, in addition to the way in which the fertilized egg develops in vitro, for the embryos which will be selected for replacement in the uterus. This approach seems to have improved the implantation rates of the embryos, but more information is necessary to establish the actual contribution of this selection to the success rate of IVF.

Carriers of a balanced reciprocal translocation or a centromeric fusion (Robertsonian translocation) have an increased risk of generating embryos, who are unbalanced (estimated at more than 80% of the fertilized eggs) and are therefore at a significant risk of developing abnormally.

FISH using probes, which identify the centromeric and the telomeric regions of the chromosome regions involved, will allow the identification of the unbalanced form of the chromosome anomaly. This approach requires the availability of probes labeled with different fluorochromes, which may not be available for all cases and therefore again requires the development of a specific and validated test.

Donor selection

In recent years, PGD has also been used in a few cases to select the best potential donor of cord blood stem cells for a sib suffering from an incurable inherited genetic disease. Not finding a compatible donor of bone marrow, the parents of a child suffering from Fanconi's anemia turned to PGD to save their child. HLA typing of the pre-embryos identified a few compatible donor embryos, which led to their implantation and the successful transplantation with cord blood stem cells of the sick sib soon after the birth of the compatible donor. Other attempts for similar indications are in progress, but few embryos are compatible donors. Combined with the limited success of PGD/IVF this does not forebode application of this approach on a large scale.

Outcome and pregnancies

The European Society for Human Reproduction and Embryology (ESHRE) has collected outcome statistics for 26 European centers. The number of clinical pregnancies out of about 1200 PGD for chromosomal anomalies or monogenic diseases is 222 (16–21%, depending on the indication). More than half of these were done for monogenic diseases. For PGD-AS the outcome is somewhat better, since 799 cycles led to 199 pregnancies (25%). Worldwide statistics show that out of more than 3000 cycles the pregnancy rate was 24%, with the same low rate of birth defects as that observed after ICSI without PGD.

Misdiagnosis

Reports about the number of misdiagnoses are limited in number. Indeed the limited number of cases, which have resulted in the birth of a child, precludes the availability of precise statistics. From the data that are available in the literature it can be estimated that the error rate is about 1–2% for DNA tested monogenic diseases, while for the misdiagnosis after blastomere biopsy and FISH for aneuploidy some studies report a 7% error rate.

Future developments

The main aim of centers providing PGD testing is to adapt and develop new methods, which will be faster, more accurate and more generally applicable than those available now.

As discussed, the application of CGH using micro arrays could be an important improvement of the accuracy and of the general applicability of the screening for any type of chromosomal anomaly. This will require that the method to amplify the whole genome will become more efficient and that the whole procedure can be automated to reduce the time necessary to arrive at a diagnosis.

For monogenetic diseases, the combination of whole genome amplification with the visualization of a series of SNPs (single nucleotide polymorphisms) in the gene which potentially carries the defect, would allow the PGD for all known monogenic diseases. Indeed, by establishing the SNP profile of the two parents around the particular gene to be tested, it would become possible to offer PGD for any known gene defect without the necessity to determine the presence of the specific molecular defect in the polar body or the blastomere. This could be done using microarrays for SNPs or by mini-sequencing of the DNA regions of interest. This would also allow the identification of contamination with exogenous DNA and would detect cases of allele-drop out.

These basic tools are available and need only to be adapted to the particular situation of PGD, making it likely that in the coming years this development will indeed find its way into the procedure.

Some PGD for diseases of the adult and for susceptibility to develop such diseases in adult life has already been offered to a few couples. This is, in particular, the case for Familial Polyposis Coli (FAP) and for hereditary forms of breast/ovarian cancer. The main difference with diseases such as Huntington's chorea for which no treatment exists is that some form, be it not fully curative, of treatment exists for these diseases and that in particular for breast cancer, the risk to develop the cancer will never be higher than 80%. The main argument to offer this PGD is that even in FAP, after removal of the colon whereby the risk for developing cancer substantially decreases, a substantial risk remains that other organs may develop cancers. The same argument exists for breast cancer. To some, this is the beginning of a slippery slope, which will end in designer babies. For others, appropriate regulation of the indications and careful counseling of the parents will never lead to such excesses.

Either way, a careful evaluation of the advantage of offering these indications, combined with a societal debate of these issues, will be the only way to provide the appropriate quality of service these couples deserve.

In conclusion

In the 15 years since PGD was shown to be a possible alternative to classic prenatal diagnosis, the successes of the procedure are undisputable. Nevertheless, the procedure remains experimental and rather exceptional. Due to technical limitations PGD has to be almost tailored to the individual case, which makes the preparatory phase expensive and time consuming. The number of cases remains limited, making an in-depth evaluation of the success rate difficult. Nevertheless, it can be expected that the technical hurdles will, in time, be removed. This will make the procedure accessible to many more couples. It might result in the first place in new approaches to determine embryo viability by FISH or CGH in all cases of IVF. Improved methods will also have an impact on the discarding of viable and normal embryos now missed by the failing technology. The main obstacle to make this the procedure of choice above classic prenatal diagnosis will probably be the inconveniences of the IVF procedure. Much will also depend on whether prenatal diagnosis, based on the analysis of fetal DNA in maternal blood, could be further developed to an almost routine procedure in the next few years. Also, the increased knowledge gained on embryonic and adult stem cells might make many aspects of PGD obsolete. Oocytes could be obtained from somatic cells or stem cells, compatible donor cells could be produced from the child's own corrected bone marrow stem cells, etc.

Authorities have a responsibility to guarantee that the procedures are of the highest quality and that the special status of the human embryo is protected. In Belgium, such a law has existed since 2003. In other countries, such as the UK, a special committee supervises the application of PGD.

In any case, it is clear that whatever the progress made in PGD, it will continue to require careful and in-depth counseling of the couples. It is indeed imperative that the couples understand what the procedure entails, what the possibilities and limitations are and that no procedure, however sophisticated it might be, will ever be able to guarantee the birth of a beautiful, healthy and intelligent child.

Further reading

K. Sermon et al. *Lancet*; 363:1633–1641, 2004.
D. Wells. Eur. *J Obstet. Gynec. Reprod.Biol.*; 115S:S97–S101, 2004.
J. Grace. *BJOG*; 11:1165–1173, 2004.
J. Schenker. *Ann N.Y Acad. Sci.*; 997:11–21, 2003.

37. Minimally invasive procedures rekindle invasive fetal therapy

Jan Deprest and Franço!s Luks, K.U.Leuven, Belgium

Introduction

Today, modern ultrasound equipment and the wide implementation of screening programmes allow the timely diagnosis of many congenital anomalies. For some of these, fetal therapy (including in-utero surgery) may be a life-saving option. Although theoretically and clinically feasible, open fetal surgery was never widely accepted because of its extreme invasiveness, and the high incidence of postoperative premature labor and rupture of the fetal membranes. In the nineties, the merger of fetoscopy and advanced video-endoscopic surgery formed the basis for the concept of endoscopic fetal surgery. We review its recent history and the contribution our group has made to this field. In 1993, the Center for Surgical Technologies of the Faculty of Medicine initiated a research program to evaluate the opportunities of fetal endoscopic ("fetendo") surgery, with the development of a unique fetal lamb model. We later demonstrated, in the non-human primate, that in-utero endoscopy is less invasive, and leads to a lesser degree of uterine activity than hysterotomy. In the late nineties, the European Commission sponsored an international project, "Eurofetus," allowing the development of a wide range of instruments by a consortium of leading clinical centers in collaboration with the medical industry. Thanks to this investment we could move from the animal laboratory to clinical practice. The first human indications for fetoscopic surgery were interventions on the umbilical cord and the

placenta – often referred to as obstetrical endoscopy. In 1995, Nico-
laides and Ville modified endoscopic laser coagulation of the placenta
in cases of previable twin-to-twin transfusion syndrome (TTTS) to
become a completely percutaneous procedure utilizing a single 3 mm
diameter cannula. In 1996, we performed the first fetoscopic cord ligation in Europe, unaware of the first successful case in the United
States performed only a few months earlier. Eurofoetus also initiated
clinical initiatives, such as a maternal safety registry and observational
studies whereby major European centers reported their experience
with obstetrical endoscopy. Thanks to this initiative, fetoscopic interventions for complicated or abnormal monochorionic twin gestations
are no longer considered experimental in Europe. Today, the outcome
of a randomized clinical trial, demonstrating that fetoscopic laser
coagulation of chorionic plate vessels is the most effective treatment
for TTTS, has revived the interest in endoscopic fetal therapy.

Clinical fetal surgery programs were non-existing in Europe until
minimally invasive fetoscopic surgery allowed operations on the
fetus to be clinically possible and acceptable from a maternal viewpoint as well. It took us seven years of animal experimentation before
performing the first clinical fetal tracheal occlusion as a therapy for
severe congenital diaphragmatic hernia. Only two years later,
promising results with this procedure could be published by a European consortium on a series of over 25 patients. As in other fields,
minimally invasive surgery has pushed back boundaries, and now
allows safe operations to be performed on the fetal patient. It offers
new hope to fetuses who are diagnosed with severe congenital malformations, and who cannot wait for treatment until after birth.
However, its further development and evaluation should follow the
strict guidelines formulated years ago for open surgery by the International Fetal Medicine and Surgery Society. Whereas minimal access
seems to solve the problem of preterm labor, all procedures remain
invasive, and carry a risk to the mother and a substantial risk of
preterm prelabor rupture of the membranes (PPROM). This problem
may prove to be a bottleneck for further developments, although
treatment modalities are currently being evaluated. Fetoscopy is technically a very challenging enterprise requiring highly specialized
equipment and skills, with a limited number of eligible patients, its
inherent potential complications and proven learning curves. There
is a need for registration and follow up of cases, so that the quality
(and number) of centers offering this modality can be controlled.

Prenatal diagnosis and screening makes the fetus a patient

The introduction of high-resolution ultrasound dramatically changed modern obstetrics. The unborn fetus became a true patient who could be directly assessed by non-invasive means. Ultrasound has become a widely implemented diagnostic tool offered to pregnant mothers in the Western world. As a consequence, information is obtained that may sometimes prompt difficult decisions by the expectant parents. Prenatal programs that screen for some incurable conditions, such as Down's syndrome, have paradoxically received more attention and financial resources than the diagnosis of conditions for which prenatal treatment may directly benefit the fetus and its parents. When fetal malformations, genetic diseases or in-utero acquired conditions are suspected, patients are ideally referred to tertiary care units with more specialized skills, technical equipment, experience and multidisciplinary counsellors who will outline potential options. In some cases, the consensus may be that intervention before birth is desirable. Sometimes, this may be offered without any direct access to the fetus, such as the administration of drugs to the mother, so that it can reach the fetus through the placenta. This has become widely accepted, e.g. in cases of cardiac arrhythmias. Other conditions, however, can only be treated by direct and invasive access to the uterus and fetus. A major breakthrough in fetal medicine was the feasibility of in-utero transfusion of the anemic fetus, first described in 1961. The procedure requires direct sampling and injection into the vascular compartment of the fetus. Today, it can be offered safely and with good fetal and long-term outcome, provided advanced skills and proper ultrasound hardware are available. Therefore, most mothers as well as their clinicians would not hesitate to seek such therapy.

Surgical conditions during intrauterine life

Many fetal conditions are amenable to surgical correction. The vast majority of these are best managed after birth; whereby sometimes, it is advisable to transfer perinatal care to a tertiary treatment center, allowing planned delivery and neonatal surgery in the same institution offering all modalities and expertise. In a limited number of conditions, however, only an in-utero intervention may save the life of the fetus or prevent permanent damage. This can be achieved

Table 37.1 Criteria for Fetal Surgery (adapted from Harrison 1991)

1. Accurate diagnosis and staging possible, with exclusion of associated anomalies
2. Natural history of the disease is documented, and prognosis established.
3. Currently no effective postnatal therapy.
4. In utero surgery proven feasible in animal models, reversing deleterious effects of the condition.
5. Interventions performed in specialised multidisciplinary fetal treatment centres within strict protocols and approval of the local Ethics Committee or I.R.B. with informed consent of the mother or parents.

by correcting the malformation, by arresting the progression of the disease, or by treating some of the immediately life-threatening effects of the condition, delaying more definitive repair until after birth. A consensus, endorsed by the International Fetal Medicine and Surgery Society (IFMSS), has been reached on the criteria and indications for fetal surgery (Table 37.1). The major challenges in applying these criteria are: (1) how to define criteria for patient selection, i.e. which fetus needs immediate intervention, which fetus can wait (until after birth) and which fetus is likely to be beyond help; (2) how to develop relevant animal models and techniques; (3) how to create multidisciplinary teams and define the legal and ethical ramifications of fetal surgery, including guidelines for counseling, informed consent and perioperative management; (4) who can offer these surgical procedures with minimal maternal and fetal risks, including the preservation of maternal fertility. This aspect of fetal medicine navigates a narrow path between potential benefits and harm to the pregnant mother and the fetal patient. Therefore, fetal surgery is not yet to be considered standard treatment, and should only be conducted in a limited number of centers of excellence.

In the 1980–90s, only a few conditions met these criteria, such as lower urinary tract obstruction, congenital diaphragmatic hernia, large space-occupying lesions of the thorax and sacrococcygeal teratoma. In the unusual situation where prenatal surgical intervention was indicated, it required maternal laparotomy, partial exteriorization of the fetus through a hysterotomy and postoperative admission of the mother to an intensive care unit. Such "open" procedures were associated with high fetal, and significant maternal morbidity, prompting the question whether the potential benefits outweighed the risks. The first open fetal operation was performed in San Francisco, in 1982, by Professor M. Harrison and colleagues, who created a vesicostomy in a fetus with obstructive uropathy. For years, and with the exception of a brief experience in Paris, open fetal surgery has been mainly an American entreprise.

In recent years, our understanding of the pathophysiology and natural history of many diseases has improved, and surgical access methods and techniques have been refined. As a result, there has been an impetus to expand the list of indications for fetal surgery, from lethal conditions to congenital anomalies that would otherwise lead to significant morbidity in the survivors. The best example is myelomeningocoele, which is not a life-threatening anomaly that can be very successfully managed after birth. However, the potential benefit from in-utero repair is to alter and modify the natural course and improve outcome after birth and avoid lifetime morbidity. This is currently being explored in a randomized trial in the United States. We do do not offer this procedure at present, nor do any other European groups, because of the associated risks to open access which at present do not outweigh unproven benefits. We are awaiting the results of this trial and restrict efforts to experimental work focussing on reducing the invasiveness of such procedure. In this respect several groups have shown that endoscopic coverage of the defect is feasible in lambs.

Another dramatic change was the improvement and miniaturization of surgical instrumentation, which led to the advent of minimally invasive surgery in fetal medicine. Therefore, the list of indications for fetal surgical intervention should be considered as a moving target, as prenatal diagnosis, pathophysiological insight, medical treatment and surgical technology improve. (Table 37.2) When such procedures are performed, one must be aware that the fetus also responds to noxious stimuli and is able to mount a neuroendocrine pain response as early as the second trimester. Whenever possible, therefore, fetal anesthesia or analgesia should be administered, either by transplacental or intrafetal route. The transamniotic route has not been used much, but appears promising.

Open fetal surgery is performed under general endotracheal anesthesia. The halogenated anesthetic gasses are myorelaxants and suppress uterine contractility. Extra analgesics and pancuronium can be given to the fetus to suppress the fetal stress response. The uterus is exposed by a large laparotomy and opened with surgical staples to

Table 37.2 Indications and rationale for in utero surgery on the fetus, placenta, cord or membranes. Historically, in utero treatment of hydrocephalus was attempted but abandoned. In the late nineties indications 5–6 were added; 7–9 were typical results of the introduction of fetoscopy in fetal surgery programs.

Fetal Surgery	Pathophysiology	Rationale for in utero therapy
1. Congenital diaphragmatic hernia	Pulmonary hypoplasia (space-occupying viscera)	Prevention of pulmonary hypoplasia
2. Lower urinary tract obstruction	Progressive renal damage by obstruction, and pulmonary hypoplasia by oligohydramnios	Prevention of renal failure and pulmonary hypoplasia
3. Sacrococcygeal teratoma	High-output cardiac failure by arteriovenous shunting and/or bleeding within a large tumor	Prevention of cardiac failure
4. Thoracic space-occupying lesions	Pulmonary hypoplasia (space-occupying mass); hydrops by impaired venous return (mediastinal compression)	Prevention of pulmonary hypoplasia and cardiac failure
5. Neural tube defects	Damage to exposed neural tube; chronic cerebrospinal fluid leak, leading to Arnold-Chiari malformation and hydrocephalus	Prevention of exposure of the spinal cord to amniotic fluid; restoration of CSF pressure and correction of Arnold-Chiari malformation
6. Cardiac malformations	Critcal lesions causing irreversible hypoplasia or damage	Prevention of hypoplasia, arrest of progression of damage
Surgery on the placenta, cord or membranes		
7. Chorioangioma	High output cardiac failure by arteriovenous shunting and polyhydramnios	prevention of cardiac failure and hydrops fetoplacentalis
8. Amniotic bands	Progressive constrictions causing irreversible neurological or vascular damage	prevention of amniotic band syndrome (deformities and function loss)
9. Abnormal monochorionic twinning; Twin-to-twin transfusion Fetus acardiacus	Intertwin transfusion leads to oligo-polyhydramnios sequence, hemodynamic changes; obstetrical complications (preterm labour and rupture of the membranes)	Arrest intertwin transfusion, prevention of cardiac failure and/or neurological damage including at the time of in utero death

prevent intraoperative maternal hemorrhage. The fetus is partially exposed or exteriorized and monitored, and the actual procedure is performed. Postoperative tocolysis includes ritodrine or its alternatives, magnesium sulphate and/or indomethacin. Afterwards, delivery by cesarean section is mandatory to prevent uterine rupture. The extreme invasiveness of this "open" approach has been a serious drawback for antenatal surgery. In addition to the wide incision, morbidity includes maternal side-effects of tocolytic agents, infection and amniotic leak. Preterm uterine activity remains the "Achilles' heel" of fetal surgery, even as the technical aspects of operating on such a frail patient have improved over the years.

Experimental endoscopic fetal surgery in animal models

The growing popularity of video-endoscopic surgery, combined with years of experience with fetoscopy, paved the way for the concept of endoscopic fetal surgery. The rationale was that key-hole access to the amniotic cavity would overcome some of the limiting steps in fetal surgery: (1) preterm labor, which was believed to be triggered by the large uterine incision of open fetal surgery; (2) significant maternal morbidity associated with a large laparotomy. It was the ultimate hope that fetoscopic interventions would be possible by percutaneous approach.

Animal experimental programs were first set up to develop new instruments and techniques; we and others used the ovine model for that purpose (Figure 37.1). Short, small diameter, leakproof and atraumatic cannulas were manufactured to access the amniotic cavity. In contrast with laparoscopy, the working space was not created by gas expansion (because of potential detrimental effects on the fetus or membranes), but by a warmed electrolyte (Hartmann's) solution, which had the triple advantage of preventing fetal hypothermia, dehydration and acidosis. Fetal surveillance devices were designed, including temperature probes, a custom-made pulse-oximetry probe to be placed around a fetal limb, and an amniotic pressure transducer. Initially, 2.3–4.5 mm diameter rod lens telescopes were used, but today small 0.5–2 mm diameter fibre endoscopes with increasing numbers of pixels are available. Endoscopes were also used to explore the fetal foregut, which would later prove to be clinically relevant (Figure 37.1). With a 3 mm diameter steerable endoscope, and later with a curved 1.2 mm fibrescope, the fetal trachea was explored. Additional tools,

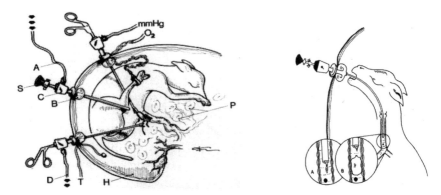

Figure 37.1 Animal models developed at the Center for Surgical Technologie at the KU Leuven. **Left:** Ovine model for fetoscopic surgery (drawing: F Luks; with permission of Am J Obstet Gynecol). Endoscopic in utero creation of lower urinary tract obstruction in the fetal lamb. Abbreviations: A=Amnioinfusion, B=Balloon, C=Cannula, D=Drainage of AmnioticFluid, H=Uterine Horn, mmHg=Pressure transducer, O2=Pulse oximitry, S=Telescope, T=Temperature probe, P=Placental cotyledons. **Right:** Endoluminal tracheal occlusion in the sheep, using one port. A catheter loaded with a balloon is inserted into the trachea (drawing: J Deprest; with permission of Ann of Surg).

such as bipolar coagulating and cutting devices and curved or articulating instruments, proved to be helpful in the special working conditions of the amniotic environment. Various fetal operations were tested, many derived from the experience in open fetal surgery or taking advantage of the scarless healing properties of the fetus. These included the creation of a lower urinary tract obstruction, dissection and ligation of the urachus, transabdominal stenting of the fetal bladder (to salvage renal function in case of urinary tract obstruction), fetoscopic repair of cleft-lip and in-utero fetoscopic covering of myelomeningocele (the latter as the basis of a subsequent clinical program). While not the primary target, many of these procedures were indeed shown to be feasible by percutaneous approach.

The ovine model is very resistant to postoperative preterm contractions, and therefore not ideal to study the most limiting factor of open fetal surgery. To test the hypothesis that endoscopic access to the uterine activity was associated with less uterine activity than after hysterotomy, we documented myometrial activity in mid-trimester rhesus monkeys (Macaca mulatta). A typical triple cannulation of the uterine cavity was made during 60 minutes. No significant postoperative premature contractions could be demonstrated, in contrast to uterine irritability following hysterotomy. Use of this higher species is limited by ethical and financial constraints, but today the model is still in use for study on healing of the fetal membranes after fetoscopic cannulation.

Fetal surgical interventions

In the next section we will focus on the indications for fetal surgery that have become clinically relevant, thanks to innovation in endoscopic or intravascular catheterization techniques. Other indications are briefly mentioned at the end.

Congenital diaphragmatic hernia

Congenital diaphragmatic hernia (CDH) affects 1 in every 2000 to 5000 babies; in just over half the cases, it is an isolated condition, not associated with chromosomal, syndromal or structural anomalies, which are independent determinants of survival. The defect does not challenge the fetus directly, but herniating viscera are believed to compete with lung development and expansion. CDH babies have smaller and less compliant lungs that have fewer airway branches, immature lung parenchyma and abnormal pulmonary vessels. Despite advances in modern neonatal care, the condition remains lethal in 30–40% of live-born babies. Improved survival rates in some series may be merely a reflection of higher termination rates in severe cases, now that the condition can be diagnosed prenatally and its prognosis established by indirect assessment of lung development. For left-sided CDH, the presence of herniation of part of the liver into the thorax and a low lung-to-head ratio (LHR) during mid-gestation are indicators of poor outcome. With an LHR <1.0 and liver herniation, there is a less than 10% chance of survival. Since postnatal care does not correct the pulmonary hypoplasia, it would seem logical to stimulate lung growth prenatally (when the placenta, rather than the lungs, are the source of gas exchange for the fetus).

Initially, surgeons emulated postnatal interventions for CDH, i.e *anatomical* repair of the diaphragm after reduction of the herniated viscera. The procedure was shown to be feasible, except when the liver was herniated, because acute reduction of the liver into the abdomen causes kinking of the ductus venosus, thereby blocking all venous (oxygen-rich) blood from the umbilical vein. Therefore the target group (severe cases are those with liver "up"), could not benefit from this fetal intervention and this approach was abandoned. As an alternative, the use of fetal tracheal occlusion (TO) was explored. TO prevents egress of lung liquid, leading to increased pulmonary stretch and accelerated lung growth which was well documented in animal models. We conducted experiments in TO for seven years, in order to find the optimal technique, timing and duration. We ultimately developed a concept of (1) percutaneous tracheoscopic intervention, with (2) endoluminal positioning of a detachable balloon with expandable properties (to accommodate tracheal growth during late gestation) and (3) reversal of obstruction before the end of gestation (plug-unplug sequence). Thus, fetoscopic endoluminal tracheal occlusion (FETO) not only avoids maternal laparotomy, hysterotomy, fetal laparotomy (for traditional repair) or neck dissection (for tracheal clipping) but also allows a normal vaginal delivery because the airways are restored prior to birth. The balloon is placed at 28 weeks under epidural anesthesia. The fetus receives fentanyl (15µg/kg) for pain relief and pancuronium (0.2 mg/kg) for immobilization by intra-muscular injection. Instruments, including a 1.2 mm diameter telescope, are passed through a 3.3 mm diameter cannula (Figure 37.2). Patients stay in hospital for two days,

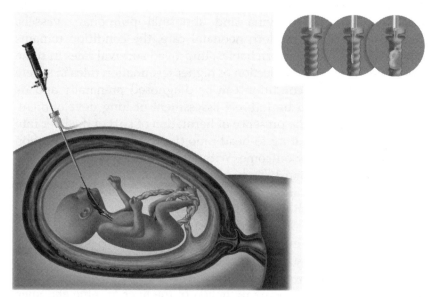

Figure 37.2 FETO procedure. A cannula is inserted in the direction of the fetal mouth. The endoscope is then advanced into the fetal pharynx and trachea. Insert: balloon deposition. (Drawings: UZ Leuven; images on the right: reprinted, with permission from International Society of Ultrasound in Obstetrics and Gynaecology and John Wiley & Sons, Ltd).

following which the lung growth is measured by ultrasound. At 34 weeks the same technique is used to retrieve the balloon; alternatively, the balloon is ruptured by ultrasound-guided needle puncture. The patients are then referred back to the tertiary referral center for postnatal management, including repair of the defect.

We have performed FETO successfully in over 35 cases now, with a mean operation time of 22 minutes. Survival rate is now 55%, compared with 8% in contemporary controls who undergo only postnatal treatment. Pulmonary morbidity is lower than expected for severe cases and survivors are not neurologically impaired at the age of one. The limiting factor of the procedure is PPROM before 32 weeks, which still occurs in 35% of cases and leads to preterm delivery in 30% of cases. This problem decreases with increasing experience, and compares favorably with numbers in an earlier trial in the US, where the procedure was done via laparotomy and 5 mm cannulation of the uterus. This shows that severe CDH may be successfully treated with minimally invasive percutaneous FETO.

Congenital heart disease

One of the most exciting areas in the field of minimally invasive fetal therapy is the treatment of congenital heart defects (CHD). Some structural defects are primarily simple, but cause a progressive abnormal development of the great vessels and ventricles, resulting in a poorly functioning heart after birth. For instance, progressive critical aortic valvular stenosis may progress to hypoplastic left heart syndrome (HLHS) and it has been speculated that in-utero reversal of the stenosis can reverse progression to ventricular hypoplasia. Currently, the only available treatment for a single-ventricle heart is staged palliative surgery (Norwood operation, followed by a Fontan procedure). The same principle may apply to progressive critical pulmonary stenosis with intact ventricular septum, which leads to hypoplasia of the right heart. There now exists some experience with ultrasound-guided fetal heart catheterization and valvular dilatation, which can often be done by percutaneous approach. The greatest experience in over 35 cases has been gathered at Harvard Medical Center in Boston, where the procedure is occasionally done by open abdomen and under general fetomaternal anesthesia. In over 50% of cases, the valvular dilatation is successful, but in about 20% of these, progression to hypoplasia cannot be reversed. Experience with HLHS with restrictive or intact atrial septum is more limited, as is that with pulmonary atresia or stenosis with intact ventricular septum. We have had limited experience with this type of intervention, but the technical aspects of it are similar to any needle-guided procedure, making it acceptable from a maternal viewpoint. However, further research will determine optimal patient selection, timing and technique for the different types of correctable heart defects.

Lower urinary tract obstruction

This sporadic condition affects 1:5000–1:8000 babies. It leads to hydro-uretero-nephrosis, renal dysplasia and pulmonary hypoplasia, result-ing either in lethal respiratory failure at birth or, for survivors, in vary-ing degrees of renal failure, requiring dialysis and/or transplantation and as a consequence of the oligohydramnios, physical deformations. The diagnosis of lower urinary tract obstruction (LUTO) can easily be made by ultrasound, typically by the presence of a dilated, thick-walled bladder, hydroureteronephrosis and oligohydramnios. Oligo-hydramnios may make structural ultrasound difficult and amnioinfu-sion should then be considered as part of the work up, next to fetal karyotyping. The exact nature of the urinary tract obstruction cannot always be determined with present diagnostic techniques; and fetoscopy may play a role in the future. Once the diagnosis is made, the degree of fetal renal function is assessed by analysis of serial fetal bladder urine samples and/or blood samples.

Electrolytes at 18–22 weks	Good renal function	Poor renal function
Sodium	<90 mmol/L	>100 mmol/L
Chloride	<80 mmol/L	>90 mmol/L
Osmolality	<180 mOsm/L	>200 mOsm/L
Calcium	<7 mg/dL	>8 mg/dL
Beta 2 microglobulin	<6 mg/L	>10 mg/L
Total protein	<20 mg/dL	>40 mg/dL

Table 37.3 Criteria for renal function as determined on serial vesicocentesis samples (Johnson et al – in Harrison M: The unborn patient; 2000.)

Occasionally, some urine can be used for rapid karyotyping. In cases where renal function is preserved, urinary deviation can prevent fur-ther renal damage. In case of poor renal function patients should be counseled likewise, but shunting may still preserve lung develop-ment. This intervention is typically done in mid-trimester, using a double pig-tail shunt (according to Rodeck), introduced by a purpose-designed trocar system. For early pregnancy there are special smaller devices available. Operative (or laser) vesicostomy has been occasionally described, but vesico-amniotic shunting by ultrasound-guided placement of a vesical stent is a more common, and well documented, procedure. The curled tail on both the bladder and the amniotic sides must prevent dislodgment and migration to the abdomen.

At present, the best documented, single hand experience is that of Johnson (Children's Hospital Philadelphia, formerly at Detroit, MI). He reviewed outcomes on 84 fetuses, who underwent evaluation by serial vesicocentesis. 49 fetuses with a good prognosis, based on the cut-offs above, survival after shunting was 75% vs. 37% in fetuses expectantly managed. In survivors who had a shunt placed, renal dysplasia occurred in 18% while in 100% of cases managed expectantly. In fetuses with poor prognosis only 6% survived, i.e. the only ones who were shunted on request of the parents, and all had renal dysplasia. In the ones dying in the neonatal period, non-shunted fetuses all had renal dysplasia, while in the ones shunted, it remained as high as 90%. The interval from shunt to delivery was 84 days; mean gestational age at delivery was 34 weeks in this series. Long-term follow-up on 78% of babies surviving till discharge is now available (mean age 5.8 years). Failure to thrive occurred in approximately 20% of cases, and 20% of survivors have pulmonary problems either limiting daily activities or sleep apnea. Forty-five percent have normal renal function, 22% mild renal insufficiency. The remaining third is on dialysis and/or is transplanted. Bladder function is normal in 61%, and one in three needs to self catheterise either permanent or intermittently.

Shunting remains an invasive procedure with a 4.8% procedure-related loss, a 40% risk for preterm labor, dislocation or obstruction of the shunt and neonatal abdominal wall defects or herniation. With the smaller so-called Harrison shunting set, dislodgment is more frequent (up to 48%) and other problems such as shunt obstruction have been described.

Fetoscopic procedures have been described, such as the creation of a vesicostomy by laser coagulation, or fetal cystoscopy and ablation of urethral valves (as in the postnatal period). This procedure is still hampered by inadequate instruments, which do not allow sufficient vision because of their size and because they cannot be directed to the bladder neck via a percutaneous approach. However, this is a clinical need. In the experience of Johnson, postnatal diagnosis of the obstruction type was highly predictive of long-term renal outcome. Posterior urethral valves do much better, while babies with urethral atresias or prune belly phenotype do less well. This underscores the belief that there is room for improvement in prenatal diagnosis and fetal cystoscopy might play an important role here.

Congenital cystic lung lesions

Congenital cystic lung lesions comprise congenital cystic adenomatoid malformations (CCAM), bronchopulmonary sequestrations and bronchogenic cysts. The common pathological mechanism for these conditions are that they act as space-occupying lesions that, if large enough, can cause pulmonary hypoplasia and/or impaired venous return, leading to hydrops fetalis. Fetal hydrops consists of subcutaneous edema, ascites and pleuro-pericardial effusions, and it is usually fatal unless treated. Many of these lesions will show impressive growth early in the second trimester, often causing mediastinal shift and compression of the ipsilateral lung. It has been proposed that the proportion size of the mass (diameter of the mass divided by head circumference, or CCAM Volume Ratio-CVR; Crombleholme) can help predict hydrops, hence fetal demise. When that ratio is greater than 1.6, there is an 80% risk of fetal hydrops. At that moment, the mother is at risk for mirror or Balentyne syndrome, particularly in the presence of placentomegaly.

The majority of lesions do not cause fetal hydrops; moreover, they will partially regress in the third trimester, and some may even be undetectable at term. Very few actually disappear, and postnatal imaging is required, even for the asymptomatic ones, because they put the child at risk of recurrent pulmonary infections and even malignancy of the persistent lesions. In 5–10% of cases, CCAMs and sequestrations may fail to regress and cause hydrops in utero. In the unlikely event of fetal hydrops over 32 weeks, management will be ex utero. The majority of cases with hydrops will present earlier and require in utero intervention. Occasionally, percutaneous puncture and thoraco-amniotic shunting of macrocystic masses may be successful, but the place of these interventions has not been well established. Laser coagulation or thermoablation of the mass has been attempted, but these techniques can cause thermal damage to surrounding structures and worsen fetal hydrops, leading to in utero death. Survivors may have skeletal chest deformation. Excision of the diseased lobes (fetal lobectomy) is possible by open fetal surgery, with good survival, as long as the hydrops resolves. In a series of 22 cases operated on between 21 and 31 weeks, there were 11 long-term survivors, who were developmentally normal (up to 12 years of age). Hydrops resolved in one to two weeks; the mediastinum shifted back more slowly, and the remaining lung showed impressive catch-up growth. Causes of fetal death despite in utero intervention were termination of pregnancy for Ballentyne syndrome (n=1), preterm labor and/or chorioamnionitis (n=2) fetal hemodynamic compromise leading to intraoperative death in six fetuses and postoperative death in another two. To prevent intraoperative deaths, all means of fetal resuscitation, including access to the fetal circulation for volume and inotropic support, and appropriate fetal monitoring techniques are now part of the open procedure.

Sacrococcygeal teratoma

Sacrococcygeal teratoma (SCT) is the most common congenital tumor (1:35,000 births). The tumor arises in the caudal cell mass of the embryonic disc, located anterior to the coccyx. It can be diagnosed as a mass as early as the first trimester. Most SCT do not require prenatal treatment and can be perfectly and functionally managed by resection after birth (survival 95%). When the SCT is larger than 5 cm, cesarean section is recommended to avoid tumor rupture and bleeding. In some cases, SCT may lead to intra-uterine high-output cardiac failure, due to the shunting effect of large arterio-venous fistulae in the tumor ("vascular steal"). Hydrops fetoplacentalis may also cause maternal symptoms, including pulmonary edema, hypertension, and proteinuria ('mirror' or Ballentyne syndrome). When the diagnosis is made prior to viability and hydrops is imminent, in utero resection may in theory benefit the fetus and the mother. Three of eight operated fetuses are reported as long-term survivors by the Fetal Treatment Center of San Francisco; there were also two postnatal losses due to malignancy and air embolism. Injection of sclerosants or fetoscopic laser or radiofrequency coagulation has been occasionally reported, but survival rates are difficult to assess. Finally, major excisional surgery in utero may result in significant structural and functional loss of the perineal body, as seen in at least one survivor.

Operative fetoscopy on the placenta, cord and membranes

Monochorionic twins

Monochorionic (MC) twins account for about 20% of twins, and 70% of identical twins. Compared with dichorionic twins, they have disproportionately high fetal loss rates, and are at higher risk for preterm delivery, perinatal mortality and morbidity. Survivors are more prone to neurologic problems, including cerebral palsy. The increased adverse outcome is mainly due to the nature of the monochorionic placenta with its unpredictable blood flow through ever-present vascular anastomoses, and its either symmetrical or asymmetrical sharing of placental mass and blood supply between the twins. Determination of chorionicity is highly accurate in the first trimester and allows early identification of these high-risk pregnancies. Therefore, these pregnancies should be followed carefully for the occurrence of well-defined complications, some of which are treatable by surgical intervention. For that reason, failure to document chorionicity in twins undergoing first trimester scanning should be considered substandard care.

Feto-Fetal Transfusion Syndrome and fetoscopic laser coagulation

In about 15% of MC twins, there is a chronic imbalance in the net flow of blood across the anastomoses, resulting in Twin Twin Transfusion Syndrome (TTTS). Hypovolemia, oliguria and oligohydramnios develop in the donor twin ("stuck twin"). Hypervolemia, polyuria and polyhydramnios are seen in the recipient twin, who often develops circulatory volume overload and hydrops. The severity of the condition correlates in part with specific patterns of vascular anastomoses, which can be identified at the surface of the placenta by fetoscopic inspection (Figure 37.3 and 37.4). The condition is diagnosed by ultrasound criteria: oliguric oligohydramnios (deepest vertical pool 2 cm) with polyuric polyhydramnios (8 cm DVP < 20 weeks; =10 cm = 20 weeks). Its natural history is not defined yet, but it is believed to be progressive, with development of abnormal Doppler patterns in the umbilical arteries of the donor fetus and/or the umbilical vein of the recipient, and ultimately fetal hydrops or fetal death. Untreated, the perinatal loss is in excess of 80% for severe cases, making therapy mandatory. Laser coagulation of chorionic plate anastomoses eliminates the underlying pathology, provided

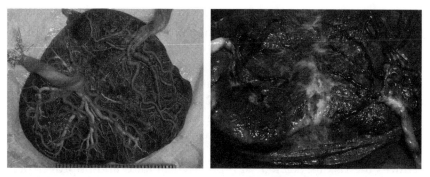

Figure 37.3 Left: injection study of a monochrorionic placenta with lasered areas (brown patches): four different colors have been used for arteries and veins from both twins. This placenta is equally shared. Right: postnatal view of a lasered placenta; white area is infarctised area of coagulation.

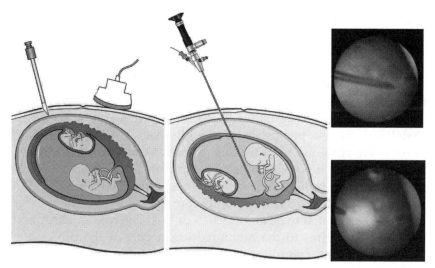

Figure 37.4 Schematic drawing of fetoscopic laser coagulation of chorionic plate vessels, in case of a posterior placenta. The trocar is first inserted percutaneously, later on a straight endoscope is inserted through the cannula. (Drawing: Katja Dalkowski; with permission from Karl Storz). Right: Fetoscopic visualisation of an arterio-venous anastomosis (top) and its coagulation (bottom) (photos: Fetal medicine unit Leuven).

that anastomosing vessels can be visualized by fetoscopy. The aim of the operation is to convert the monochorionic placenta into a functionally bi-chorionic one. For that purpose, *all* anastomoses (i.e., all vessels that connect both twins) are coagulated. The operation involves a 3 mm incision in the maternal abdomen and insertion of a 3 mm cannula, which contains a 2 mm fetoscope and 0.4 mm laser fibre (Figure 37.4). The procedure is performed by percutaneous approach and under local or loco-regional anesthesia. Amnioreduction is in itself not curative, but completes the procedure, as it reduces the risk associated with polyhydramnios and improves placental perfusion. Hospital stay is typically two days or less.

We conducted, with the Eurofoetus group, a randomized trial comparing fetoscopic laser with serial amnioreduction, which used to be the standard of care. The median gestational age at delivery was significantly higher in the laser group than in the amnioreduction group (33.3 vs. 29.0 weeks' gestation; P=0.004). Survival to 6 months of at least one twin was higher after laser (76.4% vs. 51.4%; RR=1.49; P=0.002). Amnioreduction more often led to double fetal demise (49% vs. 23%). Overall, a higher percentage of infants were alive without major neurologic morbidity at six months in the laser group. The place for amnioreduction in lower stage or early disease is currently debated, but the National Institutes of Health (NIH) trial documenting its role early on in the disease, was discontinued for a variety of reasons. New trial proposals may be launched in the future, but at present there are not many arguments to propose amniodrainage anymore.

Fetoscopic laser coagulation is the most frequently performed obstetrical endoscopic procedure, with over 1,000 registered in Europe. We currently perform this operation once or twice a week, which has made it possible to train a complete team that is available on a permanent basis. Single center series report better results than the randomized trial, but case selection may play a role. The risk for PPROM is estimated to be around 10% or less. The risk for abruption is 1–2% and relates to the amnioreduction part of the procedure. Other uncommon complications are chorioamnionitis and hemorrhage. Post-laser fetal anemia, recurrent or persistent TTTS should be screened for, and may suggest incomplete separation of the placental circulations. TTTS predisposes to right ventricular outlet tract obstruction (pulmonary stenosis) in 7% of survivors. All these conditions should be diagnosed by scrupulous postoperative ultrasound follow-up and postnatal evaluation.

Sono-endoscopic cord occlusion

Most MC twins are indeed very similar in appearance, but major dis-
cordances in structural and even in chromosomal anomalies can
occur. Abnormalities associated with twins are neural tube, brain,
facial, gastrointestinal, anterior abdominal wall and cardiac defects,
and more than 80% are discordant. An extreme form of twin discor-
dance is the twin reversed arterial perfusion sequence (TRAP). Blood
flows from an umbilical artery of the pump twin in a reversed direction into the umbilical artery of the perfused twin via a direct arte-
rio-arterial anastomosis. The perfused twin's blood supply is by definition deoxygenated and results in variable degrees of deficient
development of the head, heart and upper limb structures. The
increased burden to perfuse the parasitic twin puts the pump twin at
risk for in utero congestive heart failure and hydrops. At least 50% of
pump twins will die due to congestive heart failure or severe preterm
delivery as a consequence of polyhydramnios. When this occurs in
the previable period, intervention is mandatory. Today, the diagnosis
is made earlier, but early prediction of outcome has not been possible so far. MC twins can also be discordant for aneuploidy (trisomy
13 or 21, monosomy 45,X have been described in that respect). Counseling issues may be very difficult in heterokaryotypic twins, because
it is not possible to exclude hidden, but phenotypically important
mosaicism or microchimerism in the twin with normal karyotype.

Options for MC twin pregnancies discordant for structural and
chromosomal anomalies are expectant management, selective feticide
or termination of the entire pregnancy. There is no ethical dilemma as
to selective fetocide in case of an unviable co-twin, e.g. in TRAP
sequence, or even in TTTS complicated by severe and irreversible
anomalies. Also, when there is a high risk for in utero fetal demise
(IUFD) of one twin in the previable period, fetocide may prevent
complications to the co-twin at the moment of IUFD. In other situations the ethical dilemma is sharper. For instance, in the rare instances
of discordant chromosomal, or more commonly structural or
acquired anomalies, there is no immediate or remote risk of IUFD of
the affected fetus and, therefore, no serious threat to the other fetus.
In such situations, the predictably poor quality of life for the abnormal twin may not be acceptable to the parents, and they may not
accept the option of expectant management. In those circumstances,
selective feticide may be a more acceptable option than termination

of the entire pregnancy. The situation becomes even more complex when some of these anomalies are diagnosed very early in pregnancy, at a time when it might be impossible to reliably predict the natural history of the disease. The best example is TRAP: although the condition can be diagnosed early, not all cases lead to heart failure, polyhydramnios or IUFD of the pump twin. It is tempting to treat all such cases early on, but this approach may lead to unnecessary treatment and potential complications in some.

Conventional fetocide by intracardiac potassium chloride injection cannot be used in MC twins. In theory, this could lead to embolization to the other fetus via the ever-present anastomoses in a MC placenta, but given the amounts used that mechanism is not likely. However, the most important reason to choose other techniques is that feto-fetal hemorrhage after IUFD must be prevented. Therefore, it is recommended to arrest both arterial and venous flow in the cord of the target fetus. Historically, this was achieved by fetoscopic cord ligation, but this procedure has already been abandoned because other less complex, minimally invasive procedures have been described. Today, the best studied and most universally applicable method of cord occlusion is bipolar coagulation under sono-endoscopic guidance. Alternative techniques include the use of laser or monopolar energy.

In a prospective follow-up study of 80 consecutive cord coagulation cazes (87 fetuses), bipolar was primarily used in one-third of the cases. In the others, laser coagulation of the cord was first attempted, but in half of these cases, bipolar was necessary to arrest flow completely. The survival rate was 83%, with no difference between twins and triplets. Half of the in utero losses were in the immediate postoperative period, potentially related to incomplete occlusion (which was more likely after laser than bipolar coagulation). The other losses were thought to be due to cord complications (entanglement), an argument against creating an intertwin septostomy during the procedure. PPROM is the most common complication, and is responsible for all perinatal deaths. Seven percent of survivors exhibited abnormal psychomotor development at one year and beyond, and most of these had experienced PPROM and preterm delivery. There was a clear learning curve effect, with a dramatic decrease in PPROM and intact survival after the first 40 procedures. Therefore, we recommend that the procedures be done by an experienced operator and, wherever possible, later in gestation, to prevent the consequences of PPROM. This may not always be an option, however, because of legal and/or ethical constraints.

Ethical aspects

It is clear that fetal medicine, and especially invasive fetal procedures, with their inherent feto-maternal risk, raise ethical questions. The problem is two-fold: (1) what is the moral status of an unborn life, and (2) how do we solve the potential conflict of interest between mother and fetus? Regarding the first dilemma, one can take two extreme positions. Some ethicists base their view on the assumption that the unborn fetus is not by definition a human person with all its inherent rights, and therefore its interests could be ranked "lower" than that of the mother. If, on the other hand, the fetus is considered a person, it is endowed with human dignity and human rights, and these may deserve equal consideration with the interests of others, including the mother. This attitude discounts the fact that intrauterine life is different from life after birth. The fetus and the mother are not separate entities and the fetus is not autonomous, at least not before viability: their situation is one of interdependency in several aspects. Any intervention may have an impact on both, and should not be done if it is not in the interests of both. One cannot direct all focus on one of the two patients: if therapy only focuses on the fetus, one loses sight of the mother's interests. Conversely, if the therapy only takes maternal considerations into account, the fetal focus is forgotten. The correct attitude will not overweigh the interest of one individual over the other.

The situation for fetal therapy is even more complex, with the potential of conflict between the two individual patients. The mother has to ingest drugs, or in our case, accept an invasive intervention on herself. It is not possible to care for the fetus without "using" the mother in the process. Any intervention on the fetus can only be achieved through co-operation of the mother. The mother usually is the fetus's first, if not sole advocate and voice. At the same time, however, she must voice her own interests. Whereas in situations with double interests, we tend to consider the arguments of both sides as equal in weight, this is not necessarily so in the case of fetal therapy: here, the mother's interest seems to us to come first. The mother was individuated before the fetus came to life. The fetus derives its life from its mother, in the widest significance of the word.

It is there because she wishes it to be there, she cares for it and, before viability, it cannot exist without her. It would not even benefit from fetal medicine if it were at the expense of its mother's health.

Therefore, the mother is the primary patient in prenatal care, and any proposed intervention should be in her interest, overlapping with the fetus interest. In case of fetal intervention, there is certainly the potential for conflict: the health status of the fetus may require an unusual procedure that can harm the mother (as well as the fetus). In such a scenario, one can not expect that an intervention would be done for the fetus at the expense of the mother: it is inappropriate for fetal medicine specialists to perform even fetal life-saving procedures that would be unacceptably risky or with clinically predictable harm to the mother, even with her consent. Whereas some may argue that both fetus and mother have their own status, with their own mind, personality, rights and wishes – that is, both are moral beings – it is obvious to us that in this interdependent state, no procedure could be forced on the mother. The autonomy of the mother cannot be harmed, even if it is to save the fetus. It is the pregnant mother who confers the status of patient to her fetus(es) before viability.

Therefore, it is our moral obligation to combine minimal harm to the mother with sufficiently documented potential benefits to the pregnancy, and the fetus. This is why fetal surgery has to go through the motions of extensive animal experimentation, providing sufficient evidence of potential benefit, and allowing technical improvements to minimize maternal trauma or risk to the fetus, for example, by reducing the risk of preterm birth. That is why patients should be referred to centers with experienced teams, and anyone should refrain from embarking lightly on such programs. As to the informed consent from mothers regarding potential benefits, it is our duty to document the results of such programs. Maternal safety is a primary responsibility, but pregnancy outcomes and long-term follow-up are prerequisistes for appropriate information to future patients.

The situation of multiple pregnancy is even more complex, with several fetuses to be considered in the equation. The conditions described above do not compare with the situation of embryo reduction, since one of the fetuses is affected by a condition that is incompatible with life, or the affected fetus poses a threat to the normal twin. In those situations, procedures are performed in the vital interest of the healthy twin, and fetocide may be morally preferable to termination of the entire pregnancy. The object of fetal care is the pregnant mother and her entire pregnancy and progeny but, if due to an intrinsic disease, one fetus has a condition that does not allow it to survive, in some cases it may become a threat to the other twin. Fetocide in this instance does not place the affected fetus in a lesser moral status, but has the interest of the entire pregnancy and its outcome as the ultimate goal. On the other hand, one cannot impose this on the mother: if the mother wishes to accept the malformed fetus, even if it is a threat to the other one, we cannot force therapy on her. The most we can (and should) do is raise the arguments and voice the needs of the other (unaffected) fetus; but no intervention can be done against her will, whatever limited invasiveness it might involve.

Conclusion

In conclusion, fetoscopy has given fetal surgical therapy a new stimulus, and minimal access techniques have made it a viable option for expectaut parents. However, its application is restricted to very specific indications and experienced hands. Patients should be part of prospective follow-up programs to document case selection and the efficacy of the intervention. Fetoscopy may become a technique which will allow new therapies, such as organ-targetted gene-therapy, or may be supported by robotic surgery in more complex operations on the fetus. Since they are invasive, these procedures will always carry a substantial risk of PPROM, which is as yet an unsolved clinical problem. Therefore, our current research efforts are directed to this problem, as well as to medical therapeutical alternatives to surgery for selected fetal diseases.

Further reading

Ethical issues in fetal surgery research. Chervenak F, Mc Cullough L, Birnbach D. *Best Practice & Research Clinical Anesthesiology.* 2004; 18: 221–230.

Anesthesia for fetal intervention and surgery. Myers L, Bulich LA (Eds). BC Decker Publishers, Hamilton, 2005.

Obstetric Endoscopy. J Deprest & Y Ville. In: *The unborn patient: the art and science of fetal therapy.* M Harrison, M Evans, NS Adzick, W Holzgreve, Eds. WB Saunders Publishers, 2000, Chapter 15: 213–232.

Twin to twin transfusion syndrome. Lewi L, Dennes WJB, Fisk NM, Deprest J. In: *Fetal Medicine* (J Van Vught, L Schulman; Eds). M Dekker Publishers, 2006, in press.

Fetoscopic instrumentation and techniques. Deprest J, Barki G, Lewi L, Jani J, van Schoubroeck D, Gallot D, Spelzini F, Bueschle S, Vandevelde M, Devlieger R, Gratacos E. In: Fetal Medicine (J Van Vught, L Schulman; Eds). M Dekker Publishers, 2006, in press.

Percutaneous Fetal Endoscopic Tracheal Occlusion (FETO) for severe left sided congenital diaphragmatic hernia. J Deprest, J. Jani, E. Gratacos, H Vandecruys, G Naulaers, J Delgado, A Greenough, K Nicolaïdes, and the FETO task group. *Sem Perinatol*, 2005; 29:94–103.

A randomized trial of endoscopic laser surgery versus serial amnioreduction for severe twin-to-twin transfusion syndrome at midgestation. Senat MV, Deprest J, Boulvain M, Paupe A, Winer N, Ville Y. *New Engl J Med*. 2004, 351:136–144.

Monochorionic diamniotic twins: diagnosis and management options. Lewi L, Van Schoubroeck D, Gratacos E, Witters I, Timmerman D, Deprest J. *Curr Opin Obstet Gyneco*. 2003; 15: 177–194.

Management of fetal lung lesions. Adzick NS. *Clin Perinatol*. 2003; 30: 481–492.

Perinatal management of congenital cystic lung lesions in the age of minimally invasive surgery. Truitt A, Carr S, Cassesse J, Kurkchubasche A., Tracy T., Luks F. *J Ped Surg*. 2006 (in press)

Doctoral theses at the K.U.Leuven in this field:

François Luks: A model for fetal surgery through intrauterine endoscopy.

Jan Deprest: Endoscopic Feto-placental surgery: from animal experiments to early human applications.

Veerle Evrard: Fetoscopic surgery for Congenital Diaphragmatic Hernia.

Roland Devlieger: Fetal Membrane Healing: experimental models and preventive strategies.

Liesbeth Lewi: Fetoscopic interventions in complicated monochorionic twins: towards solutions for current problems.

Acknowledgment: This is in thankful memory of the late Kamiel Vandenberghe, Professor of Obstetrics and Gynaecology, founder of the Unit of Prenatal Diagnosis and Fetal Therapy, initial promotor of my doctoral thesis (JDP) and remembered as the father of ultrasound in Obstetrics and Gynaecology in Flanders. We thank colleagues and researchers in our endoscopic fetal surgery programme (F Luks, K Peers, V Evrard, H Flageole, N Papadopulos, M Miserez, I Dumitrascu, H Yamamoto, E Gratacos, R Devlieger, K. Vanamo, L Lewi, J Jani, X Roubliova, J Wu, D Gallot, P Vaast, F Bonati, D Challis), as well as the colleagues of the Fetal and Medicine Unit (D Van Schoubroeck, I Witters, D Timmerman) and Obstetrics Unit (B Spitz, J Verhaeghe, A Van Assche, M Hanssens) and Neonatalogy Unit (H Devlieger, C Vanhole, K Allegaert, G Naulaers, A Debeer, V Cossey) making this work and our clinical programme possible. Mrs Sybille Storz is thanked for her support in granting Dr Luks's fellowship in Leuven as well as with generous support with instruments. Our work was generously supported by grants of the KU Leuven, Fonds Wetenschappelijk Onderzoek Vlaanderen, Verkennende Internationale Samenwerking (Vlaanderen), Deutsche Forschungsgesellschaft, Sophia Stichting, Europese Commmissie.

EPILOGUE

Today, few Catholic schools of medicine in the world offer modern reproductive medicine. Notable exceptions are universities in Belgium and Netherlands that have been at the forefront of new developments in reproductive medicine for more than fifty years. At these univerisities reproductive services have been developed within a framework of freedom, respect for others, care for quality, and with the support of involved physicians, ethicists and Church leaders. The underlying bio-clinical aspects and the ethical reflections, together with the challenges, risks and errors that occurred at the K.U.Leuven during this process, have been recounted in this book. This unique model, based on personalist ethics, has not taken roots at other Catholic universities outside the Low Countries. As a consequence, a deep divide now exists in clinical practice and fertility research between Catholic centers in the Low Countries and those in the rest of the world.

A silent schism?

The major question is whether a schism is silently taking place between the teachings at Catholic universities in the Low Countries and the Catholic Church? Is it significant that the Catholic University of Nijmegen recently changed its name in Radboud University Nijmegen? Some facts, although difficult to evaluate, suggest that the divide between progressive and orthodox Catholic Universities may not be as deep as would be deduced from the official line taken by the university authorities.

In general, it has not been easy to obtain accurate information on the clinical practices in reproductive centers at different Catholic universities. At some universities, access to information was limited. Despite these restrictions, we have tried to compare objectively current practices at the major centers in the world. The history of reproductive medicine at the Catholic University of Leuven was central in this book and its dark pages have not been omitted. The intention has never been to expose individuals or to attribute personal blame but to discuss openly, as one should expect from a university, the problems, risks, and dilemmas posed by modern reproductive medicine. This story, which spans more than half a century, details the challenges faced by patients, physicians, hospital authorities, and other involved parties when modern reproductive medicine that appear to be in conflict with existing Church doctrine is introduced. It is unlikely that such a history could have been written by an outsider. Indeed, at some universities there was little access to information on topics considered sensitive and at some places instructions not to contribute to or collaborate on this book came from the University Authority. The major reason appears to be a concern, if not a fear, that transparency and access to information could be damaging to the university or embarrassing for the Church hierarchy. There is no doubt that many involved in reproductive medicine at Catholic universities worldwide are troubled by a fear of open conflict with Rome.

The physician-patient relationship

The physician-patient relationship at orthodox Catholic universities may not be as strict as implied by the official rhetoric. This has been well documented in the several contributions from these centers in this book. A surprising observation is that clinical practice at both progressive and orthodox Catholic universities remains similar and is based on profound respect for human life and care for the quality of human reproduction. At most Catholic universities, the patient can discuss openly with the physician personal issues such as contraception, sterilization, prenatal diagnosis, termination of pregnancy, infertility treatment, and other aspects of reproductive medicine. At many places, appropriate treatment cannot be offered directly but arrangements are made, such as outsourcing of services or referral to other medical centers, to accommodate the patient. These physicians care and ensure that patients receive the appropriate treatment.

The ability to make local arrangements is likely to determine the sustainability of reproductive services. When there is a policy of "no such treatment under any circumstance" and no room is left for discussion or referral, patients will stay away. Obviously, under such circumstances the physicians are hindered in their professional duty of assisting patients in need of medical help. Patients requesting abortion for socio-economic reasons will not turn to an orthodox Catholic university when this service is available elsewhere. Unfortunately, a similar trend is also apparent for patients with infertility. Caring for couples with infertility has historically been a priority at academic Catholic centers but this has steadily disintegrated in recent years. By the mid-1980s, many Catholic universities had developed great expertise in infertility management and were centers of excellence for training and treatment. With the introduction of IVF in the 1980s, and the Church opposition to this technique, patient numbers declined. As a result, those centers that adhere strictly to the Church directives have today lost the ability to provide optimal treatment for many infertile couples.

The disintegration of fertility services has two major consequences. Firstly, the ethical issues raised by the introduction of new reproductive technologies are no longer addressed or openly discussed. A second, long-term effect is that academic staff members at conservative Catholic universities lose interest in reproductive research and, consequently, are no longer at the forefront of one of the most rapidly changing disciplines in modern medicine.

It is hard to understand why Catholic universities do no offer IVF services. For patients with tubal infertility reconstructive tubal surgery remains the only acceptable treatment, even when the disease is severe. Surgery increases the risk of a tubal pregnancy without much improving the chance of a normal pregnancy. While IVF is highly effective in achieving an intrauterine pregnancy in patients with tubal disease this approach has also its own medical and ethical problems. The main medical risk is that of multiple pregnancies and the associated maternal and neonatal morbidity. The ethical dilemma of what to do with spare embryos is still unresolved. However, both problems can and will be resolved through continuing medical research. The risk of multiple pregnancies is already significantly reduced as a consequence of successful research on the efficacy of single embryo transfer. Advances in vitrification technology promise to make routine egg cryostorage a reality. The problem of spare embryos is likely to be resolved in the near future by improved protocols for ovarian stimulation, minimal use of gonadotropins, and by cryopreservation of excess oocytes rather than embryos. This raises the possibility that only a limited number of oocytes are thawed and fertilized at any one time to achieve a single or double embryo transfer. Will all this make IVF tomorrow more acceptable at orthodox Catholic schools of medicine? Should research aimed at eliminating the problem of multiple pregnancies and spare embryos not have been a priority for Catholic universities? Should the development of clinical services that improve the quality of the beginning of life not be a common goal at all Catholic universities?

A slippery slope?

Reproductive technologies are today an integral part of clinical practice and research at progressive Catholic universities in the Low Countries. All aspects of reproductive medicine are covered at these universities. The difference in practice between Catholic and other Universities in the Low Countries has not been investigated in this book. Although clinical services are likely to be more restrictive and differently orientated, the approach taken by progressive Catholic universities has resulted in a personalized and trustful patient-physician relationship and efficient clinical services. Ethical guidelines for clinical practice and research are continuously discussed and updated. Research at these centers is currently internationally competitive and focussed on prevention of reproductive disorders, understanding human reproductive ecology, and improving the quality and outcome of pregnancy.

Yet other Catholic universities worldwide have not adopted this model of reproductive medicine. A dangerous and ambivalent situation is created when a clinical service developed that is perceived to be in conflict with official Catholic doctrine. Even at the K.U.Leuven, the response has too often been to maintain discretion at all costs and, on some occasions, to impose secrecy in an attempt to avoid publicity and the risk of embarrassing the Church hierarchy. This culture of secrecy has proven to be detrimental on many occasions for patients, physicians, researchers and the university itself. As a senior member of the Academic Board of the K.U.Leuven commented after the attempt to conceal an IVF blunder was revealed: "cover-up never pays off".

The fear of embarking on a slippery slope has been a major concern for the Medical Ethics Committee at the K.U.Leuven and, consequently, its recommendations have often lacked consistency. Several examples illustrate how attempts to comply with official doctrine have caused confusion, sometimes at the expense of best clinical care.

- The Medical Ethics Committee approved the use of insemination with donor sperm when it was introduced into clinical practice in 1975. The decision, however, was not taken unanimously and remained controversial. In 1998, the Committee recommended that donor insemination should no longer be performed unless ICSI had failed. While it is justified in introducing a new technique as part of clinical research, the insistence that ICSI had to replace donor insemination was puzzling as there were no experimental or clinical data available at that time regarding the safety of this new technology.

- Egg donation, unlike sperm donation, is seen as an act of solidarity. The Committee proposed that the egg donor should be told that the risks are small, thereby trivializing the risks associated with ovarian hyperstimulation and ovum retrieval in healthy, fertile women. Death as a consequence of oocyte donation has been reported and there are no large, prospective studies on the morbidity and mortality associated with IVF treatment to prove the absence of major risks.

- In 1998, the Committee issued the stern warning that PGD leads "without any doubt" to the selection and elimination of human embryos. On the other hand, the Committee recognizes that the primary aim of PGD is to avoid invasive prenatal diagnosis and abortion of fetuses affected by incurable diseases or major degenerative disorders.

- Another example is the changing recommendation on how to manage spare embryos. Initially, the Committee was very concerned and instructed that the survival of every embryo should be a high priority. The Committee advocated IVF treatment in unstimulated, natural cycles what in practice turned out to be entirely unrealistic. Limiting the number of eggs that should be fertilized was also not acceptable as selection of the egg with the best chance of fertilization is not feasible. Therefore, the Committee suggested that when three or more eggs are fertilized, three or even four embryos should be transferred to the womb and the remainder cryopreserved for later usage. The Committee later recognized that this advice was far from satisfactory as it posed an obvious clinical dilemma. Either up to four embryos are transferred with a view to decrease the number of spare embryos or, alternatively, one or maximally two embryos are replaced with the primary aim to reduce the enormous health burden associated with multiple pregnancies. Today, priority is given to reduce the number of embryos transfered and to reduce the incidence of multiple pregnancies.

- The fact that spare embryos can now be used for research purposes will be interpreted by many as further evidence that the K.U.Leuven has embarked on a slippery slope that ultimately will lead to a total abandonment of the Christian principles that governed reproductive medicine and sciences at Catholic universities. In 1985, the Medical Ethics Committee proclaimed that, under no circumstances, could spare human embryos be used for research or their life span be extended in the laboratory longer than needed. However, in 2002 the same Committee allowed couples to donate spare embryos for stemcell research and sanctioned the culturing of thawed spare embryos to the blastocyst stage. From these blastocysts, stemcells can be obtained for experimental research. Most extraordinary of all, the Committee also allowed the donation of spare embryos to a commercial spin-off company associated with the K.U.Leuven. Contributing couples are not considered to be stakeholders and have to sign a disclaimer waiving their rights to financial compensation.

In clinical practice there have been important safeguards against a slippery slope. The ethical issues raised by modern reproductive technologies were, from the beginning, the subject of interdisciplinary dialogue. In the 1950s and 1960s, the introduction of family planning was a consequence of intensive dialogue between University and Church, as described in Chapter VIII. In the early 1970s, members of the interdisciplinary infertility team discussed the implementation of new treatments such as donor insemination and IVF. These discussions and guidelines were published in 1976 by De Wachter and collaborators in the book *Menselijke vruchtbaarheid en geboortenplanning: het paar en zijn begeleidend team* (Human fertility and birth control: the couple and its team). The Faculty of Medicine established, in 1975, a Committee for Medical Ethics that provided a series of guidelines on donor insemination (1975, 1989, 1998), in vitro fertilization (1984), abortion (1989, 1990) and preimplantation genetic diagnosis (1998). These guidelines were published in 2000 by Vermylen and Schotsmans in a book entitled *Ethiek in de Kliniek* (Ethics in the Clinic). The publication of ethical guidelines on reproductive medicine by a Catholic school of medicine is unique. Unfortunately, there is no English version but these guidelines have been extensively quoted in this book.

A common purpose

The review of research topics confirms that Catholic medical schools, whether conservative or progressive, have focussed their efforts on improving the quality of human reproduction. **Chapter X** presents a scientific anthology which is typical for the research orientation in reproductive medicine at Catholic universities.

Fertility awareness methods have not been widely accepted by the medical world as objective evidence of their efficiency has been lacking. Times are changing. Recent studies from the National Institute of Environmental Health Sciences in the US and collaborating universities have evaluated the efficacy of fertility awareness-based methods for contraception as well as for conception purposes. Today, there are major reasons to believe that teaching the body signs of fertility should be an integral part of modern reproductive medicine. Progress in human reproductive ecology depends on effective contraception as well as conception. Efficient planning of pregnancy allows the woman to optimize the environment for the implanting embryo. There is increasing evidence that the quality of the uterine microenvironment at the time of implantation and initial placentation is critical for the pregnancy outcome and future health of the offspring. The story of folic acid supplements is an impressive example that shows how fetal abnormalities can be prevented by simple manipulations at the time of conception. Conversely, the story of stilboestrol, a synthetic estrogen that was taken in early pregnancy to prevent miscarriage, is an example of how periconceptional intervention can cause permanent damage to the offspring. From the very first weeks of pregnancy, when the embryo is engaged in organogenesis, human life is vulnerable to teratogenic insults. The first two or three critical weeks of pregnancy have already passed by the time of a positive pregnancy test, further emphasizing the need for natural methods that allow effective planning of conception.

The story of fertility awareness methods illustrates how the research directions at conservative and progressive Catholic universities can be complementary and synergistic in improving the quality of reproduction. Infertility research is flourishing at progressive but not conservative Catholic universities. Conversely, research in fertility awareness is flourishing at conservative but not at progressive Catholic universities. Whatever the denomination, Catholic universities are united by their focus on improving the quality of human reproduction.

Time to leave the catacombs

In conclusion, this book is intended to contribute to a dialogue, not a divide. The book shows how modern reproductive medicine, focussed on the patient and based on Christian values, has been developed at a Catholic university by engaged physicians and ethicists during the last fifty years. However, by refusing to debate, intepret or adapt Church doctrine, other universities in the world appear to alienate a large number of couples faced with reproductive problems. As a consequence, many Catholic universities have become disengaged from the new developments in this rapidly changing field in medicine. The first step for renewed dialogue requires that Catholic universities around the world would agree to disagree on clinical practice and research in reproductive medicine without fear of upsetting the Church hierachy. Perhaps the strongest argument for openness, transparency and dialogue is the common approach taken by most Catholic physicians all over the world when treating patients with reproductive disorders. This is clearly reflected in their personal attitudes and in the shared nature of the physician-patient relationship. An understanding and appreciation for the shared goals in reproductive medicine and sciences would go a long way in bridging the current divide between Catholic universities worldwide. The opportunity to jointly and complementarily develop and shape reproductive medicine, inspired by shared christian values, during the next fifty years should not be missed.

GLOSSARY

ABORTIFACIANT AGENTS chemical substances that interrupt pregnancy after implantation

AGGIORNAMENTO Pope John XXIII called for the convocation of an Ecumenical Council of the Bishops of the Catholic Church in 1959, at the same time he called for a revision of the Code of Canon Law, that body of law which regulates the internal life of the Church. He saw these two measures as a way to awaken the Church to the human needs of the twentieth century and to open the windows of the Church to the invigorating wind of the Holy Spirit. He used the word aggiornamento to describe the renewal that he wanted to see in the Church

AID artificial insemination with donor semen

AIDS acquired immune deficiency syndrome

AIH artificial insemination by homologous (partner) sperm

AMENORRHEA not menstruating

AMNIOTIC FLUID fluid that surrounds the fetus

ANOVULATION not ovulating

ART assisted reproductive technologies

AZOOSPERMIA absence of sperm in the ejaculate

BLASTOCYST 5–7 days after fertilization, the embryo contains many cells and forms a cystic cavity within its center. At this stage, the embryo is called a "blastocyst"

CESAREAN HYSTERECTOMY surgical removal of the uterus at the time of cesarean section

CGH Comparative genome hybridization

CORPUS LUTEUM the vacated ovarian follicle that produces progesterone

CRYOPRESERVATION is freezing tissue or cells in order to preserve them for the future. Cryopreservation is used in infertility programs mainly to freeze and store sperms or to freeze "leftover" embryos from an IVF or ICSI cycle

CUMULUS MASS egg with surrounding cells at the time of ovulation

DECIDUA uterine lining modified by progesterone

DNA desoxyribonucleic acid a dimeric macromolecule that in living organs carries the genetic information

DYSMENORRHEA menstrual cramps

DYSPAREUNIA pain associated with coitus

ENDOMETRIUM uterine lining

ENDOMETRIOSIS painful disease that occurs when cells of the uterine lining (endometrium) grow somewhere in the body (usually in the pelvic cavity)

ENDOMETRIOMA a hemorrhagic cyst caused by bleeding of endometriotic cells

ESTROGEN the main female sex hormone produced by the ovary

FALOPE RING STERILIZATION Fallopian tube sterilization using small plastic rings

FIBROID a benign tumor of the uterine muscle (see MYOMA)

FISH fluorescent in situ hybridization

FOLLICLE (OVARIAN) the structure within the ovary that contains an egg and produces estrogens

FOLLICLE-STIMULATING-HORMONE (FSH) pituitary hormone that stimulates estrogen production by the ovary

GAMETES haploid cells which come together in syngamy at fertilization

GENES the 46 human chromosomes (22 pairs of autosomal chromosomes and 2 sex chromosomes) between them house almost 3 billion base pairs of DNA that contains about 30,000–40,000 protein-coding genes

GONADOTROPIN-RELEASING-HORMONE (GnRH) peptide hormone that causes the pituitary gonadotropins (LH and FSH) to be released by the ovary

GnRH-AGONIST synthetic peptide that acts like the gonadotropin-releasing hormone (GnRH)

HAPLOID CELL cell containing one set of chromosomes

HIV human immunodeficiency virus

HLA Humane Leucocyte Antigen system is the immune system that allows to distinguish between own and foreign structures

HUMAN CHORIONIC GONADOTROPIN (hCG) the placental hormone of pregnancy

HYSTERECTOMY surgical removal of the uterus

HYSTEROSALPINGOGRAPHY(HSG) an X-ray test that examines the cavity of the uterus and the patency of the Fallopian tubes

HYSTEROSCOPY endoscopic examination of the uterine cavity

ICSI intracytoplasmic sperm injection, a form of micromanipulation, involves the injection of a single sperm directly into the cytoplasm of a mature egg (oocyte) using a glass needle (pipette)

IVF in vitro fertilization is a method of assisted reproduction that involves bringing one or more eggs from a woman into contact with sperm from her partner in a laboratory dish, outside the woman's body. Usually the ovary is stimulated by hormonal medication (controlled ovarian hyperstimulation or COHS) and one or more mature eggs are aspirated using a needle from the ovary just before ovulation would occur. Once the eggs have been fertilized the resulting embryo or embryos are transferred into the womb, where it will hopefully implant in the uterine lining (endometrium) and further develop to lead to a normal pregnancy. In vitro fertilization therefore differs from in vivo fertilization in that the union of sperm and egg takes place in the laboratory, outside the woman's body

IUCD Intrauterine contraceptive device

LAPAROSCOPY surgical procedure in which an endoscope is inserted through a small incision just below the navel

LEFFSCOPE obstetrical stethoscope to listen to fetal heart beats

LUTEINIZING HORMONE (LH) pituitary hormone that stimulates the ovary and brings about ovulation

MEIOSIS the speciallized division of cells that will form sperms or eggs and reduce the chromosome number by half

MENARCHE a woman's first menstruation

MENOPAUSE the end of menstruations caused by depletion of eggs in the ovary

MICROARRAY use of DNA chips to determine which genes are activated and which genes are repressed

MITOCHONDRIA sub-cellular structure within the cytoplasm of every cell providing the energy a cell needs to move, divide, produce secretory products, contract – in short, they are the power centers of the cell.

MITOSIS the process of cell division that results in two identical daughter cells

MONAMNIOTIC TWINS twins sharing the same amniotic sac and the same placenta

MONOZYGOTIC TWINS twins derived from a single (mono) egg (zygote)

MYOMA benign fibroid tumor in the uterine muscle (see FIBROID)

MYOMETRIUM muscle layer of the uterus

NFP natural family planning

OHSS ovarian hyperstimulation syndrome

OOPHORECTOMY surgical removal of the ovaries

OVARIECTOMY surgical removal of the ovaries

PCR polymerase chain reaction

PGD preimplantation genetic diagnosis

PID pelvic inflammatory disease

PLACEBO a dummy drug or procedure used in clinical trials

POLYCYSTIC OVARY SYNDROME implies interference with the egg development and release resulting in multiple small cysts under the surface and production of higher amounts of androgens

PREMENSTRUAL SYNDROME (PMS) symptoms of physical and psychological dyscomfort before menstruation

PROGESTERONE the steroid hormone necessary to maintain pregnancy

PROLACTIN a pituitary hormone that induces lactation and prevents ovulation

PROSTAGLANDIN hormone with many bodily effects including contracting smooth muscle

PROTEOMICS measurement and characterization of plasma proteins

STROMA one of the cell types of the uterine lining

SYNGAMY the counterpart of meiosis

TRANSVAGINAL ENDOSCOPY endoscopic examination of the uterine and pelvic cavities by access through the vagina

TRANSVAGINAL HYDROLAPAROSCOPY endoscopic access examination of the pelvic cavity with access through the vagina and using saline for distension

TROPHOBLAST the membrane that surrounds the blastocyst in early development

VAS DEFERENS a tube conducting sperms from the testis to the urethra

ZYGOTE single cell embryo stage

FURTHER READING

Part 1. Bio-medical context

Chapter I, 1

Coutinho EM and Segal SJ.
Is menstruation obsolete?
Oxford, Oxford University Press, 1999.

Eaton SB, Pike MC, Short RV et al.
Women's reproductive cancers in evolutionary context.
Q Rev Biol. 1994;69:353–67.

Giudice LC, Kao LC.
Endometriosis.
Lancet. 2004;364:1789–99.

Glasier AF, Smith KB, van der Spuy ZM et al.
Amenorrhea associated with contraception – an international study on acceptability.
Contraception. 2003;67:1–8.

Missmer SA, Hankinson SE, Spiegelman D, Barbieri RL, Malspeis S, Willett WC, Hunter DJ.
Reproductive history and endometriosis among premenopausal women.
Obstet Gynecol. 2004;104:965–74.

Strassmann BI.
Menstrual cycling and breast cancer: An evolutionary perspective.
J Womens Health. 1999;8:193–202.

Treloar AE, Boynton RE, Behn BG, Brown BW.
Variation of the human menstrual cycle through reproductive life.
Int J Fertil. 1967;12:77–126.

Chapter I, 2

Bigelow JL, Dunson DB, Stanford JB, Ecochard R, Gnoth C, Colombo B.
Mucus observations in the fertile window: A better predictor of conception than timing of intercourse.
Hum Reprod. 2004;19:889–92.

Billings EL, Brown JB, Billings JJ, Burger HG.
Symptoms and hormonal changes accompanying ovulation.
Lancet. 1972;1:282–4.

Dunson DB, Baird DD, Wilcox AJ, Weinberg CR.
Day-specific probabilities of clinical pregnancy based on two studies with imperfect measures of ovulation.
Hum. Reprod. 1999; 14: 1835–9.

Dunson DB, Bigelow JL, Colombo B.
Reduced fertilization rates in older men when cervical mucus is suboptimal.
Obstet Gynecol. 2005;105:788–93.

Gnoth C, Godehardt D, Godehardt E, Frank-Herrmann P, Freundl G.
Time to pregnancy: Results of the German prospective study and impact on the management of infertility.
Hum Reprod. 2003;18:1959–66.

Gnoth C, Godehardt E, Frank-Herrmann P, Friol K, Tigges J, Freundl G.
Definition and prevalence of subfertility and infertility.
Hum Reprod. 2005;20:1144–7.

Scarpa B, Dunson DB, Colombo B.
Cervical mucus secretions on the day of intercourse: An accurate marker of highly fertile days.
Eur J Obstet Gynecol Reprod Biol. 2006;125:72–8.

Stanford JB, Smith KR, Dunson DB.
Vulvar mucus observations and the probability of pregnancy.
Obstet Gynecol. 2003;101:1285–93.

Wang X, Chen C, Wang L, Chen D, Guang W, French J.
Conception, early pregnancy loss, and time to clinical pregnancy: A population-based prospective study.
Fertil Steril. 2003;79:577–84.

Wilcox AJ, Weinberg CR, Baird DD.
Timing of sexual intercourse in relation to ovulation. Effects on the probability of conception, survival of the pregnancy, and sex of the baby.
N Engl J Med. 1995;333:1517–21.

Wilcox AJ, Baird DD, Dunson DB, McConnaughey DR, Kesner JS, Weinberg CR.
On the frequency of intercourse around ovulation: Evidence for biological influences.
Hum Reprod. 2004;19:1539–43.

Chapter I, 3

Gordts S, Campo R, Rombauts L, Brosens I.
Endoscopic visualization of the process of fimbrial ovum retrieval in the human.
Hum Reprod. 1998;13:1425–8.

Gordts S, Campo R, Brosens I.
Endoscopic visualization of oocyte release and oocyte retrieval in humans.
Reprod Biomed Online. 2002;4 Suppl 3:10–3.

Schultz WW, van Andel P, Sabelis I, Mooyaart E.
Magnetic resonance imaging of male and female genitals during coitus and female sexual arousal.
BMJ. 1999;319:1596–600.

Chapter I, 4

Brosens I, Robertson WB, Dixon HG.
The physiological response of the vessels of the placental bed to normal pregnancy.
J Pathol Bacteriol. 1967;93:569–79.

Brosens I, Robertson WB, Dixon HG.
The role of the spiral arteries in the pathogenesis of pre-eclampsia.
Obstet Gynecol Annu. 1972;1:177–91.

Brosens IA.
Morphological changes in the utero-placental bed in pregnancy hypertension.
Clin Obstet Gynaecol. 1977;4:573–93.

Brosens JJ, Pijnenborg R, Brosens IA.
The myometrial junctional zone spiral arteries in normal and abnormal pregnancies: A review of the literature.
Am J Obstet Gynecol. 2002;187:1416–23.

Pijnenborg R, Dixon G, Robertson WB, Brosens I.
Trophoblastic invasion of human decidua from 8 to 18 weeks of pregnancy.
Placenta. 1980;1:3–19.

Pijnenborg R, Robertson WB, Brosens I, Dixon G.
Review article: Trophoblast invasion and the establishment of haemochorial placentation in man and laboratory animals.
Placenta. 1981;2:71–91.

Pijnenborg R, Bland JM, Robertson WB, Brosens I.
Uteroplacental arterial changes related to interstitial trophoblast migration in early human pregnancy.
Placenta. 1983;4:397–413.

Pijnenborg R, Bland JM, Robertson WB, Dixon G, Brosens I.
The pattern of interstitial trophoblastic invasion of the myometrium in early human pregnancy.
Placenta. 1981;2:303–16.

Ramsey EM, Houston ML, Harris JW.
Interactions of the trophoblast and maternal tissues in three closely related primate species.
Am J Obstet Gynecol. 1976;124:647–52.

Chapter II, 5

Baird DD, Newbold R.
Prenatal diethylstilbestrol (DES) exposure is associated with uterine leiomyoma development.
Reprod Toxicol. 2005;20:81–4.

Kaufmann P, Black S, Huppertz B.
Endovascular trophoblast invasion: Implications for the pathogenesis of intrauterine growth retardation and pre-eclampsia.
Biol Reprod. 2003;69:1–7.

Missmer SA, Hankinson SE, Spiegelman D, Barbieri RL, Michels KB, Hunter DJ.
In utero exposures and the incidence of endometriosis.
Fertil Steril. 2004;82:1501–8.

Chapter II, 6

Eriksson JG.
The fetal origins hypothesis – 10 years on.
BMJ. 2005;330:1096–7.

Holemans K, Aerts L, Van Assche FA.
Lifetime consequences of abnormal fetal pancreatic development.
J Physiol. 2003;547:11–20.

Nathanielsz PW.
Life in the Womb: The Origin of Health and Disease.
Promethean Press, Ithaca, New York, 1999.

Chapter II, 7

Sallmen M, Weinberg CR, Baird DD, Lindbohm ML, Wilcox AJ.
Has Human Fertility Declined Over Time?: Why We May Never Know.
Epidemiology. 2005;16:494–9.

te Velde ER.
Zijn emancipatie en voortplanting nog met elkaar te combineren in deze eeuw?
Rede uitgesproken vrijdag 19 maart 2004 ter gelegenheid van het afscheid als hoogleraar Voortplantingsgeneeskunde, Rijksuniversiteit te Utrecht.

Chapter III, 8

Akande VA, Hunt LP, Cahill DJ, Jenkins JM.
Differences in time to natural conception between women with unexplained infertility and infertile women with minor endometriosis.
Hum Reprod. 2004;19:96–103.

Duijkers I, Engels L, Klipping C.
Length of the menstrual cycle after discontinuation of oral contraceptives.
Gynecol Endocrinol. 2005;20:74–9.

Dunson DB, Colombo B, Baird DD.
Changes with age in the level and duration of fertility in the menstrual cycle.
Hum Reprod. 2002;17:1399–403.

Fédération CECOS, Schwartz D, Mayaux MJ.
Female fecundity as a function of age: Results of artificial insemination in 2193 nulliparous women with azoospermic husbands.
N. Engl. J. Med. 2982; 306, 404–6.

Gnoth C, Frank-Herrmann P, Schmoll A, Godehardt E, Freundl G.
Cycle characteristics after discontinuation of oral contraceptives.
Gynecol Endocrinol. 2002;16:307–17.

Habbema JDF, Collins J, Leridon H, Evers JLH, Lunenfeld B, teVelde ER.
Towards less confusing terminology in reproductive medicine: A proposal.
Hum Reprod. 2004; 19, 1497–501.

Hanafi MM.
Factors affecting the pregnancy rate after microsurgical reversal of tubal ligation.
Fertil Steril. 2003;80:434–40.

Olive DL, Lindheim SR, Pritts EA.
Endometriosis and infertility: What do we do for each stage?
Curr Womens Health Rep. 2003;3:389–94.

Chapter III, 9

Brosens I, Gordts S, Valkenburg M, Puttemans P, Campo R, Gordts S.
Investigation of the infertile couple: When is the appropriate time to explore female infertility?
Hum Reprod. 2004;19:1689–92.

Coutifaris C, Myers ER, Guzick DS et al.
Histological dating of timed endometrial biopsy tissue is not related to fertility status.
Fertil Steril. 2004;82:1264–72.

Gnoth C, Godehardt D, Godehardt E, Frank-Herrmann P, Freundl G.
Time to pregnancy: Results of the German prospective study and impact on the management of infertility.
Hum Reprod. 2003;18:1959–66.

Gnoth C, Godehardt E, Frank-Herrmann P, Friol K, Tigges J, Freundl G.
Debate continued: Definition and prevalence of subfertility and infertility.
Hum Reprod. 2005;20:1144–7.

Koninckx PR, Goddeeris PG, Lauweryns JM, de Hertogh RC, Brosens IA.
Accuracy of endometrial biopsy dating in relation to the mid-cycle luteinizing hormone peak.
Fertil Steril. 1977;28:443–5.

Koninckx PR, Heyns WJ, Corvelyn PA, Brosens IA.
Delayed onset of luteinization as a cause of infertility.
Fertil Steril. 1978;29:266–9.

McGovern PG, Myers ER, Silva S et al.
Absence of secretory endometrium after false-positive home urine luteinizing hormone testing.
Fertil Steril. 2004;82:1273–7.

National Collaborating Center for Women's and Children's Health. Fertility: Assessment and Treatment for People with Fertility Problems. Commissioned by the National Institute for Clinical Excellence.
London: RCOG Press, 2004.
http://www.nice.org.uk

Wang X, Chen C, Wang L, Chen D, Guang W, French J.
Conception, early pregnancy loss, and time to clinical pregnancy: A population-based prospective study.
Fertil Steril. 2003;79:577–84.

Chapter III, 10

Basso O, Olsen J.
Subfecundity and neonatal mortality: Longitudinal study within the Danish national birth cohort.
BMJ. 2005;330:393–4.

Chapter IV, 11

Olivius C, Friden B, Borg G, Bergh C.
Why do couples discontinue in vitro fertilization treatment? A cohort study.
Fertil Steril. 2004;81:258–61.

Schroder AK, Katalinic A, Diedrich K, Ludwig M.
Cumulative pregnancy rates and drop-out rates in a German IVF programme: 4102 cycles in 2130 patients.
Reprod Biomed Online. 2004;8:600–6.

Smeenk JM, Verhaak CM, Stolwijk AM, Kremer JA, Braat DD.
Reasons for dropout in an in vitro fertilization/intracytoplasmic sperm injection program.
Fertil Steril. 2004;81:262–8.

Chapter IV, 13

Antsaklis A, Souka AP, Daskalakis G, Papantoniou N, Koutra P, Kavalakis Y, Mesogitis S.
Embryo reduction versus expectant management in triplet pregnancies.
J Matern Fetal Neonatal Med. 2004;16:219–22.

Evans MI, Ciorica D, Britt DW.
Do reduced multiples do better?
Best Pract Res Clin Obstet Gynaecol. 2004;18:601–12.

Dodd J, Crowther C.
Multifetal pregnancy reduction of triplet and higher-order multiple pregnancies to twins.
Fertil Steril. 2004;81:1420–2.

Chapter IV, 14

Hansen M, Bower C, Milne E, de Klerk N, Kurinczuk JJ.
Assisted reproductive technologies and the risk of birth defects—a systematic review.
Hum Reprod. 2005;20:328–38.

Paoloni-Giacobino A, Chaillet JR.
Genomic imprinting and assisted reproduction.
Reprod Health. 2004;26;1:6.

Schieve LA, Meikle SF, Ferre C, Peterson HB, Jeng G, Wilcox LS.
Low and very low birth weight in infants conceived with use of assisted reproductive technology.
N Engl J Med. 2002;346:731–7.

Schieve LA, Rasmussen SA, Buck GM, Schendel DE, Reynolds MA, Wright VC.
Are children born after assisted reproductive technology at increased risk for adverse health outcomes?
Obstet Gynecol. 2004;103:1154–63.

Chapter IV, 15

Harris J.
Assisted reproductive technological blunders (ARTBs).
J Med Ethics. 2003;29:205–6.

van Kooij RJ, Peeters MF, te Velde ER.
Twins of mixed races: Consequences for Dutch IVF laboratories.
Hum Reprod. 1997;12:2585–7.

Part 2. Reproductive medicine at the Catholic University of Leuven

Chapter V, 16

Ferin J.
Artificial induction of hypo-estrogenic amenorrhea with methylestrenolone, or with lynestrenol.
Acta Endocrinol (Copenh). 1962;39:47–67.

Ferin J, Janssens L.
Progestogènes et moral conjugal.
Louvain, Publ. Univ.; Gembloux, Duculot.

Janssens L.
L'inhibition de l'ovulation est-ell moralement licite?
Ephemerides Theologiae Lovanienses, 1958.

Janssens L.
Morale conjugale et progestogènes.
Ephemerides Theologiae Lovanienses, 1963.

Chapter V, 17

Croxatto HB, Ortiz ME, Muller AL.
Mechanisms of action of emergency contraception.
Steroids. 2003;68:1095–8.

Eskes TK.
The pill is not an abortive agent.
Eur J Obstet Gynecol Reprod Biol. 1997;72:1–2.

Chapter V, 18

Brosens I, Winston R.
Reversibility of female sterilization.
Academic Press, London, 1978, 193pp.

Nijs P, Brosens I.
Reversibility of sterilization. Psych(patho)logical aspects.
Acco Leuven, 1981, 211pp.

Chapter V, 20

Steeno O.
Ik wil een kind. Een jongen? Een meisje? Is een bewuste geslachtskeuze ethisch verantwoord?
Periodiek 2001; 56, 7–16 en 43–53.

Steeno O, Adimoelja A, Steeno J.
Separation of X- and Y-bearing human spermatozoa with the sephadex gel-filtration method.
Andrologia. 1975;7:95–7.

Wilcox AJ, Weinberg CR, Baird DD.
Timing of sexual intercourse in relation to ovulation. Effects on the probability of conception, survival of the pregnancy, and sex of the baby.
N Engl J Med. 1995;333:1517–21.

PRINTED ON PERMANENT PAPER • IMPRIME SUR PAPIER PERMANENT • GEDRUKT OP DUURZAAM PAPIER - ISO 9706

N.V. PEETERS S.A., WAROTSTRAAT 50, B-3020 HERENT